The Nursing Student's Self Study Guide

Revised First Edition

Dr. Cheryl Davis, DNP, MSN, RN, CNE
Triton College

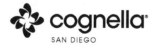

cognella®
SAN DIEGO

Bassim Hamadeh, CEO and Publisher
Angela Schultz, Senior Field Acquisitions Editor
Carrie Baarns, Manager, Revisions and Author Care
Kaela Martin, Project Editor
Rachel Kahn, Production Editor
Jess Estrella, Senior Graphic Designer
Alexa Lucido, Licensing Manager
Natalie Piccotti, Director of Marketing
Kassie Graves, Vice President of Editorial
Jamie Giganti, Director of Academic Publishing

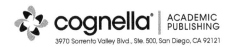

cognella® | ACADEMIC PUBLISHING
3970 Sorrento Valley Blvd., Ste. 500, San Diego, CA 92121

Dedicated to my students.

Contents

Preface

Being in nursing school is not easy. It takes commitment and perseverance. It requires you to learn material in a different way. This different way is often referred to as critical thinking. Being a critical thinker means taking concepts learned in class and developing a mental "tool kit" to solve patient problems. This mental tool kit helps you disseminate information, understand, comprehend, organize, analyze and then implement it.

Using the self study guide will assist you in organizing your studies as you listen to lecture or read your text. It is a guide to help you organize and prioritize the information on specific topics. It also will help you save time as you have one place to take your notes and also do activities to connect the concepts and understand content better.

Tidbits for nursing school success

- As you read or listen to lecture, organize the content.
- Do not be afraid to ask questions and participate in class.
- Your work on the course really begins after lecture. So review material, work with a study group or study buddy to discuss content. You are not alone in this nursing school journey and talking to someone and getting different perspectives on material is an excellent way to broaden your understanding of content.

Things to keep in mind as you study

There are foundational things you always need to remember as you learn new material. These things are:

- Your ABCs (Airway, Breathing, Circulation). … These are important when prioritizing care.
- Safety issues. Usually safety is a major priority when caring for the client.
- Always refer to Maslow's hierarchy of needs: (remembering, understanding, applying, analyzing, evaluating, and creating). Keep in mind that the client's physiological need must be first.
- Your nursing process. Remember before you can do anything for your patient, you must ASSESS. That is the first part of the nursing process.

It is my hope that this book will be a beneficial tool to help you develop a systematic way to take notes and learn material. Work hard, be committed, and good luck!!

Dr. Cheryl Davis

Electrolytes and the Role of Acid-Base and Their Part in Maintaining Homeostasis

Introduction

This chapter will examine electrolytes and the role of acid-base and their part in maintaining homeostasis.

WATER COMPRISES APPROXIMATELY 60% of the body weight of an average adult. The percentage is lower in obesity, since adipose tissue contains less water than lean tissue. It is also lower in women than in men because of the relatively greater amount of adipose tissue in women. The normal distribution of fluids varies in the different body compartments.

Minerals that carry an electrical charge when dissolved in liquid are called electrolytes. Sodium, potassium, chloride, and bicarbonate are electrolytes that are in the blood. Electrolytes help to maintain homeostasis by maintaining normal fluid levels in each fluid compartment in the body. By the process of osmosis, fluids are shifted between compartments to maintain a balance. So, if there is a high concentration of electrolytes in a compartment, fluids are moved into the compartment, and if electrolyte concentration is low, fluid moves out of that compartment. The kidneys also have a role in maintaining balances of electrolytes. They can filter electrolytes and water to and from the blood. The kidneys can also excrete excesses into the urine. If there is any imbalance in the distribution of electrolytes, disorders can develop. IV fluids are administered in some cases for patients who cannot meet their normal fluid or electrolyte levels.

Blood has a degree of acidity or alkalinity. This is indicated by the pH scale. Ranges of the scale are 0 (strong acid) to 14 (strong alkaline or base). If the pH is neutral, it is at 7.0; pH is based on levels of carbon dioxide and bicarbonate, which are acids and bases in the blood.

Learning Objectives of This Section

Upon completion of this chapter, the student should be able to:

- Discuss the pathophysiology and clinical manifestations of fluid/electrolyte/acid/base problems.
- Define terms associated with fluid/electrolyte/acid/base problems.
- Differentiate the normal and abnormal data of physical assessment of fluid/electrolyte/acid/base problems.
- Describe diagnostic test for fluid/electrolyte/acid/base problems.
- Describe common health-related fluid/electrolyte/acid/base problems.

- Describe the process involved in maintaining normal fluid and electrolyte balance.
- Describe the process and implement a nursing care plan to treat fluid/electrolyte/acid/base problems.
- Describe the pharmacological agents for fluid/electrolyte/acid/base problems.

Section I. Fluid/Electrolytes

Case Scenario 1: A 35-year-old client presents to the emergency department with complaints of vomiting and diarrhea for the last two days. He states he ate some leftovers he brought home from a birthday party. The client is admitted and diagnosed with gastroenteritis.

Lab results reveal the following: Na+ 125mEq/L; K+ 2.8mEq/L; Cl- 92mEq/L.

The health care provider has placed the client on NPO with advance as tolerated diet after the nausea and vomiting have subsided. Strict I & O. Intravenous fluids of 0.9% normal saline at 100mL/hr have been ordered.

Self Study Guide

COMPLETE THE FOLLOWING as you listen to the lecture and/or refer to your textbook.

1. Name fluid compartments within the body and the major electrolytes within each.

_____

_____

_____

_____

_____

_____

_____

_____

2. What is the purpose of intravenous therapy?

_____

_____

_____

_____

_____

_____

3. Define *tonicity*.

_____

_____

_____

_____

_____

_____

_____

4. Differentiate between *osmolality* and *osmolarity*.

_____
_____
_____
_____
_____
_____
_____
_____

5. Name the different types of IV solutions and their purpose.

_____
_____
_____
_____
_____
_____
_____
_____

6. What are electrolytes? What are they responsible for?

_____
_____
_____
_____
_____
_____
_____
_____

7. Describe the different mechanisms of movement.

_____
_____
_____
_____
_____
_____
_____
_____

8. How is water balance regulated?

_____

_____

_____

_____

_____

_____

_____

List the normal values for the adult client for the following electrolytes:

1. Sodium (Na+) =   _____

2. Potassium (K+) =   _____

3. Chloride (Cl-) =   _____

4. Calcium (Ca+) =   _____

5. Phosphate (PO4) = _____

6. Magnesium (Mg+) = _____

Significance of Sodium

_____

_____

_____

_____

_____

Normal Value

_____

Sources of Sodium

_____

_____

_____

_____

_____

Control of Sodium

_____

_____

_____
_____
_____

Functions of Sodium

_____
_____
_____
_____
_____

Alterations in Sodium Balance: Hypernatremia and Hyponatremia

Hypernatremia

Define:

_____
_____
_____
_____
_____

Causes:

_____
_____
_____
_____
_____

Diagnostic Findings

_____
_____
_____

Medical Management

_____
_____
_____
_____
_____

Nursing Management

_____
_____
_____
_____
_____
_____

Signs and Symptoms

_____
_____
_____
_____
_____
_____

Hyponatremia

Define:

_____
_____
_____
_____
_____
_____

Causes:

_____
_____
_____
_____
_____
_____

Diagnostic Findings

_____
_____
_____

Medical Management

_____
_____
_____
_____
_____

Nursing Management

_____
_____
_____
_____
_____

Signs and Symptoms

_____
_____
_____
_____
_____

Significance of Potassium

_____
_____
_____
_____
_____

> **Tidbit**
>
> Intravenous potassium (KCl) should never exceed a rate of 10mEq/hr as it can cause cardiac arrest.

Normal Value

_____

Sources of Potassium

_____
_____
_____
_____
_____

Control of Potassium

_____
_____
_____
_____
_____

Functions of Potassium

_____
_____

_____
_____
_____

Alterations in Potassium Balance: Hyperkalemia and Hypokalemia

Hyperkalemia

Define:

_____
_____
_____
_____
_____

Causes:

_____
_____
_____
_____
_____

Diagnostic Findings

_____
_____
_____

Medical Management

_____
_____
_____
_____
_____

Nursing Management

_____
_____
_____
_____
_____

Signs and Symptoms

_____

_____

_____

_____

_____

Hypokalemia

Define:

_____

_____

_____

_____

_____

Causes:

_____

_____

_____

_____

_____

Diagnostic Findings

_____

_____

_____

Medical Management

_____

_____

_____

_____

_____

Nursing Management

_____

_____

_____

_____

_____

Signs and Symptoms

_____
_____
_____
_____
_____
_____

Significance of Calcium

_____
_____
_____
_____
_____
_____

Tidbit

Calcium levels are regulated primarily by the parathyroid gland and vitamin D.

Normal Value

_____

Sources of Calcium

_____
_____
_____

Control of Calcium

_____
_____
_____
_____
_____

Functions of Calcium

_____
_____
_____
_____
_____

Alterations in Calcium Balance: Hypercalcemia and Hypocalcemia

Hypercalcemia

Define:

_____
_____
_____
_____
_____
_____

Causes:

_____
_____
_____

Diagnostic Findings

_____
_____
_____

Medical Management

_____
_____
_____
_____
_____

Nursing Management

_____
_____
_____
_____
_____

Signs and Symptoms

_____
_____
_____
_____
_____

Hypocalcemia

Define:

_____
_____
_____
_____
_____

Causes:

_____
_____
_____
_____
_____

Diagnostic Findings

_____
_____
_____

Medical Management

_____
_____
_____
_____
_____

Nursing Management

_____
_____
_____
_____
_____

Signs and Symptoms

_____
_____
_____
_____
_____

Significance of Phosphate

_____

_____

_____

_____

_____

Normal Value

_____

Sources of Phosphate

_____

_____

_____

_____

_____

Control of Phosphate

_____

_____

_____

Functions of Phosphate

_____

_____

_____

_____

_____

Alterations in Phosphate Balance: Hyperphosphatemia and Hypophosphatemia

Hyperphosphatemia

Define:

_____

_____

_____

_____

_____

Causes:

_____
_____
_____
_____
_____

Diagnostic Findings

_____
_____
_____

Medical Management

_____
_____
_____
_____
_____

Nursing Management

_____
_____
_____
_____
_____

Signs and Symptoms

_____
_____
_____
_____
_____

Hypophosphatemia

Define:

_____
_____
_____
_____
_____

Causes:

_____

_____

_____

_____

_____

Diagnostic Findings

_____

_____

_____

Medical Management

_____

_____

_____

_____

_____

Nursing Management

_____

_____

_____

_____

_____

Signs and Symptoms

_____

_____

_____

_____

_____

Significance of Magnesium

_____

_____

_____

_____

_____

Tidbit

Urine magnesium levels will show a deficiency in magnesium before serum magnesium levels will.

Normal Value

_____

Sources of Magnesium

_____
_____
_____
_____
_____

Control of Magnesium

_____
_____
_____
_____
_____

Functions of Magnesium

_____
_____
_____

Alterations in Magnesium Balance: Hypermagnesium and Hypomagnesium

Hypermagnesium

Define:

_____
_____
_____
_____
_____

Causes:

_____
_____
_____
_____
_____

Diagnostic Findings

_____
_____
_____

Medical Management

_____
_____
_____
_____
_____

Nursing Management

_____
_____
_____
_____
_____

Signs and Symptoms

_____
_____
_____
_____
_____

Hypomagnesium

Define:

_____
_____
_____
_____
_____

Causes:

_____
_____
_____
_____
_____

Diagnostic Findings

_____
_____
_____

Medical Management

_____
_____
_____
_____
_____

Nursing Management

_____
_____
_____
_____
_____

Signs and Symptoms

_____
_____
_____
_____
_____

Section I. Application Exercise 1

Review the case scenario at the beginning of the chapter. Are the client's lab results normal or abnormal? List the major clinical signs and symptoms for the abnormal values.

Electrolyte	Abnormal Value	Major Clinical Signs/Symptoms

Section I: Application Exercise 2

The vomiting and diarrhea in the client have stopped. The client has now been placed on a clear liquid diet. The Unlicensed Assistive Personnel (UAP) has recorded the 24 hr I & O for the client. The results are:

IV Fluids	=	2200	Emesis	=	800
Oral	=	130	Diarrhea	=	750
			Urine	=	660
Total	=	2330	Total	=	2210

Based on the client's I & O record, select the most appropriate nursing diagnosis for the client and develop interventions for the diagnosis:

_____ Excess fluid volume

_____ Risk for injury

_____ Imbalanced nutrition: More than body requirements

_____ Deficient fluid volume

_____ Diarrhea

_____ Imbalanced nutrition: Less than body requirements

_____ Impaired skin integrity

Nursing Interventions	Rationale

Section II. Acid Base

Case Scenario 2: A 57-year-old client is seen by the health care provider. She is complaining of chest pain and shortness of breath. The client states she feels as if she has gained weight and has some bilateral edema to her lower extremities. Her history reveals that she has chronic kidney disease, GERD, and osteoporosis. Lab results indicate low potassium (2.5) and a pH of 7.55, pCO_2 of 50mmHg, and bicarbonate of 45mEq/L.

Acid Base

Define:

_____
_____
_____
_____
_____

Normal acid-base ratio:

_____
_____
_____

Control of Acid-Base System:

1st Response

_____
_____
_____
_____
_____

2nd Response

_____
_____
_____
_____
_____

3rd Response

_____
_____
_____
_____
_____

Acidosis

Define:

_____

_____
_____
_____

Respiratory Acidosis

Define

_____
_____
_____

Causes

_____
_____

Compensation

_____
_____

Diagnostic Findings

_____
_____
_____

Signs and Symptoms

_____
_____
_____
_____
_____

Medical Management

_____
_____
_____
_____
_____

Nursing Management

_____
_____
_____
_____
_____

Metabolic Acidosis

Define

_____
_____
_____

Causes

_____
_____

Compensation

_____
_____

Diagnostic Findings

_____
_____
_____

Signs and Symptoms

_____
_____
_____
_____
_____

Medical Management

_____
_____
_____
_____
_____

Nursing Management

_____
_____
_____
_____
_____

Section II. Application Exercise

What type of acid-base imbalance is the patient exhibiting? What role does the low potassium play in this imbalance?

Answer:

_____
_____
_____

Alkalosis

Define:

_____
_____
_____
_____
_____

Respiratory Alkalosis

Define

_____
_____
_____

Causes

_____
_____

Compensation

_____
_____

Diagnostic Findings

_____
_____
_____

Signs and Symptoms

_____
_____
_____
_____
_____

Medical Management

_____
_____
_____
_____
_____

Nursing Management

_____
_____
_____
_____
_____

Metabolic Alkalosis

Define

_____
_____
_____

Causes

_____
_____

Compensation

_____
_____

Diagnostic Findings

_____

_____

_____

Signs and Symptoms

_____

_____

_____

_____

_____

Medical Management

_____

_____

_____

_____

_____

Nursing Management

_____

_____

_____

_____

_____

Section III. Purpose of Blood Gases

A blood gas test measures the amount of oxygen and carbon dioxide in the blood. It may also be used to determine the pH of the blood, or how acidic it is. The test is commonly known as a blood gas analysis or arterial blood gas (ABG) test. A blood gas test provides a precise measurement of the oxygen and carbon dioxide levels in the body. This can help the health care provider determine how well the lungs and kidneys are working. Identifying imbalances in the pH and blood gas levels can also help the health care provider monitor treatment for certain conditions, such as lung and kidney diseases.

Interpreting Blood Gas Values (Tic-Tac-Toe and ROME Mnemonic)

Tic-Tac-Toe Method

When you are analyzing ABG results, there are three things to look for when trying to find out if your patient is in respiratory or metabolic acidosis or alkalosis. Here they are, and their normal numeric values (commit them to memory):

- pH: 7.35–7.45
- CO_2: 35–45 (CO_2 lab value ALWAYS indicates a RESPIRATORY issue)
- HCO_3: 22–26 (HCO_3 lab value ALWAYS indicates a METABOLIC issue)

Now to determine when these values are considered an acid or base. For pH, anything less than 7.35 is an acid and anything greater than 7.45 is a base. For CO_2 (note: it is the opposite), anything less than 35 is a base and anything greater than 45 is an acid. For HCO_3, anything less than 22 is an acid and anything greater than 26 is a base. Here is a guide to help you understand it:

	Acid	Normal	Base
pH	7.35		7.45
CO_2	45		35
HCO_3	22		26

Let's talk about blood pH for a moment because if FULL compensation presents, there will NOT be a tic-tac-toe, and you will have to look closely at the blood pH to determine which system is causing the issue and which system is trying to "fix" the issue (hence compensate).

A normal blood pH is 7.35–7.45. The absolute normal is 7.40. Any normal blood pH that falls between 7.35–7.40 is NORMAL but on the "acidotic" side, and any normal blood pH that falls between 7.40–7.45 is on the "alkalotic" side.

In order to use the tic-tac-toe method, you must first get a sheet of paper and set up a tic-tac-toe grid. Then label each column as "acid," "pH," and "base." It should look like this:

Acid	Normal	Base

Now let's solve a problem using the tic-tac-toe method: ABG results are the following ... pH 7.24, PCO_2 75, HCO_3 28.

1. Draw your tic-tac-toe layout.

2. Analyze your pH. Ask yourself: is it normal, basic, or acidic? Since the pH is less than 7.35, making it an acid, place it under the Acid column.

3. Analyze your PCO_2. Ask yourself: is it normal, basic, or acidic? Since the PCO_2 is greater than 45, making it an acid, place it under the Acid column along with pH. Remember, PCO_2 is the opposite, and the normal is 35–45.

4. Analyze your HCO_3. Ask yourself: is it normal, basic, or acidic? Since HCO_3 is greater than 26, making it basic, place it under the Base column because the value is considered basic.

5. Your tic-tac-toe layout should look like this:

Acid	Normal	Base
pH		HCO_3
PCO_2		

Now that you have your tic-tac-toe grid set up, you need to figure out what you have. Since your pH is acidic, you know that you have acidosis going on, but is it respiratory or metabolic acidosis? Since CO_2 represents respiratory and it is under the Acid column, with your pH you have respiratory acidosis going on.

But is it fully compensated, partially compensated, or uncompensated respiratory acidosis? Look at your HCO_3! Since your HCO_3 is under basic, the metabolic system is trying to balance the body's system by becoming basic, so it is partially compensating. So the answer is Partially Compensated Respiratory Acidosis. Note: If HCO_3 was under the Normal column, it would not be trying to compensate, and therefore it would be considered uncompensated respiratory acidosis.

Section III. Application Exercise 1

Let's try another problem: blood pH 7.37, $PaCO_2$ 33, and HCO_3 17 … tic-tac-toe should look like this:

Acid	Normal	Base
HCO_3	pH	$PaCO_2$

Pull again from your memory bank to analyze the values. You should determine this:

pH: 7.37 (falls within 7.35–7.45) = NORMAL, but it's on the acidotic side

$PaCO_2$: 33 (less than 35) = ALKALOTIC

HCO_3: 17 (less than 22) = ACIDIC

So, we don't have a tic-tac-toe; therefore, the values are representing compensation (is it partial or full?).

To determine the type of compensation, look at the pH … is it normal or abnormal? It's NORMAL! Therefore, we have full compensation.

BUT is this a respiratory or metabolic problem?

To determine this, look at the blood pH:

The blood pH is normal, but it falls on the acidotic side. Our metabolic system is also acidotic, but our respiratory system is alkalotic. The problem is with the metabolic system, and the respiratory system is trying to balance out the blood's acidotic state by decreasing the carbon dioxide level ($PaCO_2$) to make things more alkaline, which will help increase the blood's pH from its acidotic state … which it has, and this is why we have full compensation rather than partial. Note: If the pH was not normal and the HCO_3 was still acidotic, it would be partial compensation. On the flip side, if the pH was not normal but the HCO_3 was normal, it would be uncompensated.

Our answer is: **metabolic acidosis, fully compensated by the means of respiratory alkalosis.**

ROME Mnemonic

You only need to really memorize 2 values: **35–45 and 22–26 (since the normal pH is 7.35–7.45 and the normal PCO_2 = 35–45).**

Next, you need to know the following Acronym: **ROME**

a. **R**espiratory = **O**pposite

b. **M**etabolic = **E**qual

Next, you want to draw a small chart and label it as indicated below:

	PCO$_2$	HCO$_3$
Acid ↓		
Alka ↑		

When presented with an acid base imbalance question, first you will look at your pH value. If the pH is lower than normal, this would indicate = ACIDOSIS. If the pH is higher than normal, this would indicate = ALKALOSIS. Once you have determined if the value represents Acidosis or Alkalosis, circle the indicator on the chart or cross out the nonrelevant value. For example, a **pH of 7.31 would indicate ACIDOSIS**; therefore, the alkalosis component of the chart is crossed off.

	PCO$_2$	HCO$_3$
Acid ↓	↓	Normal
~~Alka ↑~~		

Now you insert your values, and note with arrows the direction of any abnormal values. For example, if the PCO$_2$ was lower than the normal value (lower than 35), you would place a DOWN arrow in the CO$_2$ box. **Values: pH = 7.31 PCO$_2$ = 30 HCO$_3$ = 24.**

	PCO$_2$	HCO$_3$
Acid ↓	↓	Normal
~~Alka ↑~~		

Finally, you compare the direction of the arrows using the acronym ROME!

a. Respiratory = Opposite

b. Metabolic = Equal

Always compare the arrow in the PCO$_2$-HCO$_3$ vs. the arrow in the direction of the pH. So, in the above scenario, you would compare the DOWN-facing arrow of the pH (ACIDIC) with the DOWN-facing arrow of the PCO$_2$ (since the value was LOWER than normal). Because the values go in EQUAL directions, you have a METABOLIC disorder. Therefore, the above scenario represents METABOLIC ACIDOSIS!!

Compensated Acid-Base Imbalance Using ROME

Whenever possible, the body will try and correct the acid-base imbalance by compensatory mechanisms. For example, if a person was experiencing metabolic acidosis, the respiratory system might try to compensate by blowing off CO$_2$ (which is highly acidic) to remove acid from the system.

A value is considered partially compensated when the pH is still abnormal.

A value is considered fully compensated when the pH returns within a normal value.

Let's look at the below scenario: pH: 7.48 PCO$_2$: 25 HCO$_3$: 20.

First: Determine if this is Acidosis or Alkalosis.

Second: Place the arrows regarding high or low values for PCO_2 and HCO_3 in the appropriate boxes.

	PCO₂	HCO₃
~~Acid~~ ↓		
Alka ↑	↓	↓

1. You are looking at an elevated pH, indicating ALKALOSIS.

2. Next, look at the PCO_2; this would indicate a LOWER-than-normal value.

3. Next, look at the HCO_3; this would also indicate a LOWER-than-normal value.

Go back to the ROME acronym.

Remember, you are comparing the direction of the pH arrow (which indicates acidosis or alkalosis) with the direction of the other arrow. In this scenario, both the PCO_2 and the HCO_3 arrows face down, indicating there is some level of compensation occurring in the body.

Note: The arrow of the pH and the PCO_2/ HCO_3 go in OPPOSITE directions.

Answer: RESPIRATORY ALKALOSIS with partial compensation.

Section III. Application Exercise 2

Acid-Base Concept Map: Using the word list provided, fill in the concept map. This will assist you in better understanding acid-base balance.

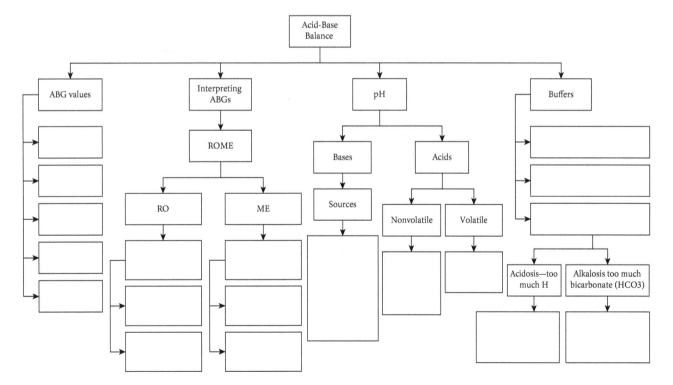

Word List for Concept Map

> pH is down, HCO_3 is down, metabolic acidosis
>
> PaO_2 80–100
>
> pH is up and HCO_3 is up, metabolic alkalosis
>
> Base Excess + 2
>
> Lungs act within minutes—hypo- or hyperventilation
>
> If pH and HCO_3 go in same direction, metabolic
>
> If pH and CO_2 are opposite, respiratory
>
> $PaCO_2$ 35–45mmHg
>
> Chemical acts within seconds
>
> Reabsorb bicarbonate ions back into blood instead of excreting them into the urine
>
> pH 7.35–7.45
>
> Bicarbonate (HCO_3) 22–26
>
> Excrete bicarbonate ions in the urine. Use ammonia mechanism
>
> Kidneys delayed (hours or days) but most powerful
>
> Bicarbonate (HCO_3)-ECF & ICF, Proteins, Hemoglobin-ICF, Albumin and Globulin-ECF. Ammonium—breakdown of amino acids
>
> Carbonic acid, excreted as a gas (lungs)
>
> pH is UP, carbon dioxide DOWN—respiratory alkalosis
>
> pH is DOWN, CO_2 is UP—respiratory acidosis
>
> Phosphoric, lactic acid, sulfuric excreted from the body in water (kidney)

Critical Thinking Questions

1. The health care provider has prescribed 40mEq/L IV potassium chloride (KCl) for treatment of a client with severe hypokalemia. Which action should the nurse take?

    a. Administer the KCl as a rapid IV bolus.

    b. Infuse the KCl at a rate of 10 mEq/hour.

    c. Only give the KCl through a central venous line.

    d. Discontinue cardiac monitoring during the infusion.

2. The client has a diagnosis of hyponatremia. A solution of 3% NaCl IV has been prescribed. Which assessment is **most** important for the nurse to monitor for while the patient is receiving this infusion?

    a. Lung sounds

    b. Urinary output

    c. Peripheral pulses

    d. Peripheral edema

3. A client presents to the emergency department with lethargy and deep, rapid respirations. The following arterial blood gas (ABG) results are: pH 7.32, PaO_2 88 mm/Hg, $PaCO_2$ 37 mm/Hg, and HCO_3 16 mEq/L. What acid-base status is the client experiencing?

   a. Metabolic acidosis

   b. Metabolic alkalosis

   c. Respiratory acidosis

   d. Respiratory alkalosis

4. A nurse on the unit is monitoring a client who has a magnesium level of 1.3 mg/dL. Which assessment would be **most** important for the nurse to make?

   a. Daily alcohol intake

   b. Intake of dietary protein

   c. Multivitamin/mineral use

   d. Use of over-the-counter (OTC) laxatives

5. Using the tic-tac-toe method or ROME mnemonic, determine the acid base state of the client. Lab values: pH 7.56, $PaCO_2$ 20, HCO_3 20:

   a. respiratory alkalosis, uncompensated

   b. respiratory alkalosis, uncompensated

   c. respiratory alkalosis, partially compensated

   d. metabolic alkalosis, partially compensated

References

Intravenous Fluid Therapy: Intravenous Fluid Therapy in Adults in Hospital [Internet] (2013, December). Retrieved from: https://www.ncbi.nlm.nih.gov/books/NBK333103/

Lewis III, J. L. (2019). Overview of acid-base balance. Retrieved from: http://www.primededucation.ca/wp-content/uploads/2014/11/ROME-Method-for-Acid-Base-Imbalance.pdf

Lewis, S. L., Dirksen, S. R., & Heitkemper, M. M. (2014). Test Bank. Medical-surgical nursing: Assessment and management of clinical problems. 9th ed. Mosby-Elsevier.

PRIMED Educational Associates Easy Guide to Acid Base Computation (2019). Retrieved from http://www.primededucation.ca/wp-content/uploads/2014/11/ROME-Method-for-Acid-Base-Imbalance.pdf

RegisteredNurseRN.com (2019). (Arterial Blood Gas.) Practice Quizzes with Tic Tac Toe Method. Retrieved from: https://www.registered-nursern.com/abg-arterial-blood-gas-practice-quizzes-with-tic-tac-toe-method/

Chapter 2

Oxygenation and Alterations in the Respiratory System

Introduction

This chapter will look at oxygenation and alterations in the respiratory system.

T HE RESPIRATORY SYSTEM begins at the nose and mouth and passes down to the pharynx and larynx. The larynx is covered with the epiglottis, which closes during swallowing and prevents food from entering the airways.

The taking in of oxygen and eliminating carbon dioxide is the primary role of the respiratory system. As the body inhales oxygen, it enters the lungs and reaches the alveoli. The exchange of gases takes place at this level of the alveoli and capillaries. There are three processes that are required for oxygen to be transferred from outside air into the blood flowing through the lungs. These processes are:

- Ventilation: process of moving air into and out of the lungs;
- Diffusion: the movement of gases between the gas at the alveoli level and the capillaries in the lungs;
- Perfusion: the pumping of blood by the cardiovascular system to the lungs.

The diaphragm controls the work of breathing (inhalation and expiration), along with the muscles between the ribs, neck, and abdomen. This is a passive process. The lungs and chest wall are elastic. They actively stretch during inhalation and return to a resting shape to exhale or expel out air in the lungs during relaxation. During activity, the body's abdominal muscles are activated and push the diaphragm against the lungs and air is pushed out. The contraction of muscles for breathing is also dependent on the nerves connecting them to the brain. If there is an injury such as a motor vehicle accident or trauma, the connection is lost between the nervous system, brain, and muscles, and death can occur.

Learning Objectives for This Chapter

Upon completion of this chapter, the student should be able to:

- Discuss the pathophysiology and clinical manifestations of the patient with selected respiratory system alterations of transportation.
- Define terms associated with the respiratory transportation system.

- Differentiate the normal and abnormal data of physical assessment of the respiratory ventilation system.
- Describe oxygen therapy and the different delivery systems.
- Describe diagnostic tests for respiratory perfusion system alterations.
- Describe common upper and lower respiratory health problems.
- Describe respiratory failure in adult patients.
- Describe respiratory age-related changes in upper and lower respiratory systems.
- Describe the process and implement a nursing care plan to treat upper and lower respiratory alterations.
- Describe the pharmacological agents for upper and lower respiratory system alterations.
- Identify chest percussion and vibration, positioning in the orthopneic position, teaching diaphragmatic and pursed-lip breathing.
- Identify and perform the steps involved in positioning for postural drainage.

Section I. Chronic Obstructive Pulmonary Disease

Case Scenario: A 74-year-old-man presents to the health care provider's office with his wife, complaining of shortness of breath and fever. His current symptoms include the following:

- Unable to speak in full sentences for the past several hours per wife.
- Cough productive but unknown color of sputum.
- Audible wheezing since last night per wife.
- Mild chest tightness.
- Dyspnea.
- His wife states that the client usually has a cough that is worse in the morning with production of gray sputum. She states that he gets short of breath if he walks more than 10 feet and has episodes of wheezing if he gets sick (e.g., with an upper respiratory infection).
- He usually can help around the house with light work and fixing things.

Vital Signs: BP: 128/74; P: 68, reg; RR: 32; Ht: 5ft 6 in; Wt: 122 lbs; T: 101.5°F oral.

Self Study Guide

COMPLETE THE FOLLOWING as you listen to the lecture and/or refer to your textbook:

Chronic Obstructive Pulmonary Disease (COPD)

Define:

_____

_____

_____

_____

Etiology/Pathophysiology

Risk Factors:

_____
_____
_____
_____

Emphysema:

Define:

_____
_____
_____
_____
_____

Chronic Bronchitis:

Define:

_____
_____
_____
_____

Clinical Manifestations:

_____
_____
_____
_____

Barrel Chest:

Define:

_____
_____
_____
_____

Tripod Position:

Define:

_____
_____
_____
_____

Section I. Application Exercise 1

Look at the data from the previous scenario. What other data would be needed for your assessment? List them here.

_____
_____
_____

Study Results

- Pulse oximetry 86%
- Chest X-ray shows hyperinflation and right lower lobe pneumonia

The client has been diagnosed with chronic obstructive pulmonary disease (COPD) and pneumonia. Should the client be treated on an outpatient basis or be hospitalized? _____
What determined your answer?

_____
_____
_____

COPD Classification:

FEV1: Define

_____
_____
_____
_____

FVC: Define

_____
_____
_____
_____

Classification	Level of Severity	FEV1 Results
Gold 1		
Gold 2		
Gold 3		
Gold 4		

Section I. Application Exercise 2

What stage of COPD using the GOLD criteria does this client have? Describe why.

_____

Complications of COPD

Cor Pulmonale:

Define:

_____
_____
_____
_____

Diagnostic Studies:

_____
_____
_____
_____

COPD Exacerbation:

Define:

_____
_____
_____
_____

Treatment:

_____
_____
_____
_____

Section I. Application Exercise 3

Hospital Course

During hospitalization, he receives the following treatment:

- Nebulized albuterol/ipratropium every 4 hrs as needed
- Prednisone 60 mg daily by mouth
- 1 gm IV ceftriaxone plus 500 mg oral azithromycin daily
- Oxygen to maintain PO2 > 60 mmHg

What is the purpose of the prescribed regimen?

_____

_____

_____

_____

Preparation for Discharge

- Over 3 days, the client has significantly improved and has been placed on an oxygen regimen of 2 liters via nasal cannula.
- He is taking the albuterol/ipratropium nebulized treatments every 6 hrs and is ready to switch back to bronchodilators via inhaler device.
- Along with antibiotics for a total of 7 days, you need to determine the dose and duration of treatment for oral corticosteroids.
- In completing the medication reconciliation forms, you see that the client had a complex medication regimen upon admission.
- It is clear during discussions with him that he is unable to comply with this expensive, complex, and potentially unnecessary regimen.

Develop a discharge care plan to meet the medication regimen for the client.

Nursing Diagnosis	Client Goals	Interventions

Section II. Acute Respiratory Failure

Case Scenario: A COPD client presents to the emergency department with rapid, shallow breathing. He states he has a bad cold and has been congested for the last few days. Temperature is 99.6 and respirations are 26. He is slumped over and states he can breathe better this way. He is restless and agitated. He is only able to communicate with two- or three-word sentences. He is given 2 liters of O_2 via nasal cannula and is admitted to the unit with Acute Respiratory Failure.

Acute Respiratory Failure:

Define:

_____
_____
_____
_____

Hypoxemic Respiratory Failure:

Define:

_____
_____

Hypercapnic Respiratory Failure:

Define:

_____
_____
_____
_____

Clinical Manifestations:

_____
_____
_____
_____

Section II. Application Exercise 1

Match the diagnostic studies done for the patient with Respiratory Distress.

Diagnostic Studies	Purpose
A. Arterial Blood Gases	Necessary to determine sources of infection___
B. Chest X-ray	Monitors oxygenation status___
C. Pulse Oximetry	Visualizes possible causes of respiratory failure___
D. Sputum/Blood Cultures	Can detect pulmonary embolism___
E. Lung/CT Scan	Determines $PaCO_2$ levels, PaO_2, Bicarbonate, and pH___

Section II. Application Exercise 2

The client's tests reveal that the acute respiratory distress is due to pneumonia. Determine some nursing interventions related to the following nursing diagnosis:

- Impaired Gas Exchange
- Ineffective Airway Clearance
- Ineffective Breathing Pattern

Interventions

Respiratory Therapy	Drug Therapy	Nutrition

Section III. Oxygen Therapy

Case Scenario: The client presents to the emergency department with complaints of shortness of breath. He stated this happened when he was chased by a dog. The client is anxious but is responding appropriately to your questions.

His vital signs are: P: 110, R: 33, SpO_2: 88%.

Oxygen Therapy:

Uses:

_____

_____

_____

_____

Methods of delivery and nursing interventions:

1. Face Mask

    _____
    _____
    _____
    _____

2. Nasal Cannula

    _____
    _____
    _____
    _____

3. Partial Non-Rebreather Mask

    _____
    _____
    _____
    _____

4. Oyxgen-Conserving Mask

    _____
    _____
    _____
    _____

5. Tracheostomy Collar

    _____
    _____
    _____
    _____

6. Venturi Mask

    _____
    _____
    _____
    _____

7. High-Flow Nasal Cannula

_____
_____
_____
_____

Humidification/Nebulization:

_____
_____
_____
_____

Section III. Application Exercise 1

From the previous scenario, what would you do for this patient?

_____
_____
_____

Complication of O_2 Use

Combustion:

_____
_____
_____
_____

O_2 Narcosis:

_____
_____
_____
_____

O_2 Toxicity:

_____
_____
_____
_____

Infection:

_____
_____

_____
_____

Section III. Application Exercise 2

What will you teach the client about O_2 therapy?

_____
_____
_____
_____

Section IV. Respiratory Interventions

Breathing Retraining:

Purpose:

_____
_____

Pursed-Lip Breathing:

Define:

_____
_____
_____
_____

Diaphragmatic Breathing:

Define:

_____
_____
_____
_____

Effective Coughing:

Purpose:

_____
_____

> *Tidbit*
>
> Clients cannot necessarily change their lung capacity in terms of how much oxygen their lungs can hold. It is important to teach them how to perform exercises that may reduce shortness of breath when they have a lower lung function. People with COPD are prime examples of this.

Huffing Coughing:

Define:

_____
_____
_____
_____

Chest Physiotherapy:

Purpose:

_____
_____

Percussion:

Define:

_____
_____
_____
_____

Vibration:

Define:

_____
_____
_____
_____

Postural Drainage:

Define:

_____
_____
_____
_____

Section IV. Application Exercise

Develop a Plan of Care for the client with COPD.

Nursing Management:

<u>Assessment: Subjective Data</u>

_____
_____
_____
_____
_____
_____
_____
_____
_____
_____
_____

<u>Objective Data</u>

_____
_____
_____
_____
_____
_____
_____
_____
_____
_____

<u>Nursing Diagnosis</u>

_____
_____
_____
_____
_____
_____
_____
_____
_____
_____

Planning/Implementation

_____
_____
_____
_____
_____
_____
_____
_____
_____
_____
_____
_____

Evaluation

_____
_____
_____
_____
_____
_____
_____
_____
_____
_____
_____

Critical Thinking Questions

1. Ineffective airway clearance, related to tracheobronchial obstruction or secretions, is a nursing diagnosis. Which nursing interventions are correct? *(Select all that apply.)*

    a. Offer small, frequent, high-calorie, high-protein feedings.

    b. Restrict fluid intake to decrease congestion.

    c. Encourage generous fluid intake.

    d. Have the patient turn and cough every 2 hrs.

    e. Teach effective coughing technique.

2. A client with chronic obstructive pulmonary disease (COPD) reports social isolation. What does the nurse encourage the client to do?

    a. Join a support group for people with COPD.

    b. Ask the client's physician for an antianxiety agent.

    c. Verbalize his or her thoughts and feelings.

    d. Participate in community activities.

3. What information about nutrition does the nurse teach a client with chronic obstructive pulmonary disease (COPD)? *(Select all that apply.)*

   a. Avoid drinking fluids just before and during meals.

   b. Rest before meals if you have dyspnea.

   c. Have about six small meals a day.

   d. Practice diaphragmatic breathing against resistance four times daily.

   e. Eat high-fiber foods to promote gastric emptying.

   f. Eat dry foods rather than wet foods, which are heavier.

   g. Increase carbohydrate intake for energy.

4. The nurse is assessing a client with chronic obstructive pulmonary disease (COPD) to determine activity tolerance. Which questions elicit the most important information? *(Select all that apply.)*

   a. What color is your sputum?

   b. Do you have any difficulty sleeping?

   c. How long does it take to perform your morning routine?

   d. Do you walk upstairs every day?

   e. Have you lost any weight lately?

Section V. Pneumonia

Case Scenario: A 75-year-old client is seen in the health care provider's office with a cough and shortness of breath. He has a history of emphysema and was released from the hospital 2 days ago after undergoing a cholecystectomy. The incision site is clean and dry. He complains of feeling tired and hot. His respirations are labored and shallow. Auscultation of the lungs reveals crackles throughout right lung fields and left upper lobe, rhonchi over larger airways, and diminished breath sounds at the base of the left side.

Vital signs: BP: 142/80, P: 120, R: 26, T: 103.4, SpO2: 88%.

Orders: Chest X-ray, sputum specimen.

Chest X-ray reveals LLL pneumonia, and results of sputum reveal that the client has an infection caused by methicillin-resistant *Staphylococcus aureus* (MRSA).

Tidbit

The National Center for Health Statistics reports that older individuals are at higher risk of dying from respiratory infections.

Pneumonia

Define:

_____
_____
_____
_____

Etiology/Pathophysiology:

Causative Organisms:

Bacterial:

_____
_____
_____

Viral:

_____
_____
_____

Risk Factors:

_____
_____
_____
_____
_____
_____
_____
_____
_____
_____

Section V. Application Exercise I

From the scenario above, what are the factors that might predispose the client to pneumonia?

_____
_____
_____
_____

Three ways in which an organism reaches the lungs:

1.

_____
_____

2.

_____

3.

_____

_____

Classification of Pneumonia:

Community Acquired (CAP):

Define:

_____

_____

Medical Care Associated Acquired (MCAP):

Define:

_____

_____

Types:

_____

_____

_____

Types of Pneumonia:

Aspiration:

_____

_____

_____

_____

Opportunistic:

_____

_____

_____

_____

Clinical Manifestations:

_____

_____

_____

_____

Diagnostic Studies:

_____

_____

_____

_____

_____

_____

_____

_____

_____

_____

Complications:

_____

_____

_____

_____

_____

_____

_____

_____

_____

_____

_____

Section V. Application Exercise 2

Match the causative agents with the correct pneumonia classification.

Classification	Causative Agent
Community Acquired	Methicillin-resistant *S. Aureus*
Health Care Associated	*S. Aureus*
Hospital Acquired	*Legionella* *Escherichia Coli* *Haemophilus influenzae* *Chlamydia pneumoniae*

Nursing Management:

Assessment: Subjective Data

_____

_____

_____
_____
_____
_____
_____
_____
_____
_____
_____

Objective Data

_____
_____
_____
_____
_____
_____
_____
_____
_____
_____
_____

Nursing Diagnosis

_____
_____
_____
_____
_____
_____
_____
_____
_____
_____
_____
_____

Planning/Implementation

_____
_____
_____
_____
_____
_____
_____
_____
_____
_____
_____

Evaluation

_____
_____
_____
_____
_____
_____
_____

Critical Thinking Questions

1. The nurse assesses a client with pneumonia and notes decreased lung sounds on the left side and decreased lung expansion. What is the nurse's best action?

    a. Have the client cough and breathe deeply.

    b. Check oxygen saturation and notify the health care provider.

    c. Perform an arterial blood gas analysis.

    d. Increase oxygen flow to 10 L/min.

2. The nurse is teaching a client with pneumonia ways to clear secretions. Which intervention is the most effective?

    a. Administering an antitussive medication.

    b. Administering an antiemetic medication.

    c. Increasing fluids to 2 L/day if tolerated.

    d. Having the client cough and breathe deeply hourly.

3. A client who works in a day care facility is admitted to the emergency department. The client is diagnosed with pneumonia, and a sputum culture is taken. Infection with *Streptococcus pneumoniae* is confirmed. What is the nurse's primary action?

    a. Have emergency intubation equipment nearby.

    b. Teach the client about the treatment.

    c. Isolate the client.

    d. Perform chest physiotherapy.

4. Which person is at greatest risk for developing a community-acquired pneumonia?

    a. Middle-aged teacher who typically eats a diet of Asian food.

    b. Older adult who smokes and has a substance abuse problem.

    c. Older adult with exercise-induced wheezing.

    d. Young adult aerobics instructor who is a vegetarian.

Section VI. Tuberculosis

Case Scenario: A 50-year-old male client is brought into the emergency department by paramedics. The client states he is homeless and lives in a tent city along the highway. He has frostbite on his right toes. The client reports that he is very fatigued and eats when he can get to the local church's food pantry for meals, but lately he has not had an appetite. He says he has lost some weight and states he has some chills and sweats at night. He is immediately placed in a negative airflow isolation room.

Tuberculosis

Define:

_____

_____

_____

_____

Tidbit

The prevalence of tuberculosis has declined in the United States, but people who are homeless, IV drug users, and foreign-born individuals are at risk for developing tuberculosis (TB).

Etiology/Pathophysiology

Causative Organisms:

_____

_____

_____

_____

Classifications

Primary:

_____

_____

_____

_____

Latent:

_____

_____

_____

_____

Active:

_____

_____

_____
_____

Clinical Manifestations:

_____
_____
_____
_____
_____

Section VI. Application Exercise 1

From the previous scenario, why was the client placed in a negative airflow isolation room? What is he at risk for, and why?

_____
_____
_____
_____
_____
_____

Complications

Miliary TB:

_____
_____
_____

Pleural TB:

_____
_____
_____

Empyema:

_____
_____

Section VI. Application Exercise 2

What are some of the other screening tests that should be done for this client?

_____
_____

_____

_____

_____

Diagnostic Studies

Tuberculin Test:

_____

_____

_____

_____

_____

_____

Sputum Tests:

_____

_____

_____

_____

_____

Chest X-ray:

_____

_____

_____

_____

_____

Bronchoscopy/Bronchial Washing:

_____

_____

_____

_____

_____

Section VI. Application Exercise 3

The client's chest X-ray reveals active pulmonary tuberculosis. He has been admitted to the unit for treatment of frostbite to the right toes and treatment of TB.

Describe how tuberculosis is spread and what type of respiratory precautions should be included.

_____

_____

_____

_____

_____

_____

Medication Regimen

Isoniazid (INH):

_____

_____

_____

Rifampin:

_____

_____

_____

Pyrazinamide (PZA):

_____

_____

_____

Section VI. Application Exercise 4

After 7 days in the hospital, the client is preparing for discharge. He is given discharge instructions that include:

- Home health nurse to administer medication regimen of INH, rifampin, and pyrazinamide (PZA) twice a week for 60 days.
- He is to follow up with the health care provider for chest X-rays and sputum cultures every week for the next 3 weeks.
- Stay away from crowds and refrain from close physical contact with others for the next 2 weeks.

Create a discharge plan for the client that includes the following:

Referral:

_____

_____

_____

Client Teaching:

_____
_____
_____
_____
_____
_____

Medication Teaching:

_____
_____
_____
_____
_____

Preventing the spread of infection:

_____
_____
_____
_____
_____
_____

Nursing Management

Nursing Diagnosis

_____
_____
_____
_____
_____
_____
_____
_____
_____
_____

Planning/Implementation

_____
_____
_____
_____

_____

_____

_____

_____

_____

_____

_____

_____

Evaluation

_____

_____

_____

_____

_____

_____

_____

_____

_____

_____

Critical Thinking Questions

1. The nurse has completed the discharge instructions for the client taking rifampin. Which statement by the client indicates that further teaching is needed?

    a. I will complete taking all of the medications as prescribed.

    b. I will call the doctor if my urine and tears are orange.

    c. This drug can produce hepatitis.

    d. Kidney failure can happen with this medication.

2. The unlicensed assistive personnel (UAP) is assigned to take care of a client with active tuberculosis (TB). Which action, if performed by the UAP, would require an intervention by the nurse?

    a. The patient is offered a tissue from the box at the bedside.

    b. A surgical face mask is applied before visiting the patient.

    c. A snack is brought to the patient from the unit refrigerator.

    d. Hand washing is performed before entering the patient's room.

3. The client returns to the clinic for a follow-up visit after 2 months of being treated for tuberculosis (TB). His regimen included isoniazid (INH), rifampin, and pyrazinamide (PZA). The sputum smear collected showed a positive result for acid-fast bacilli (AFB). What is the nurse's best action to take at this time?

    a. Teach about treatment for drug-resistant TB treatment.

    b. Ask the patient whether medications have been taken as directed.

    c. Schedule the patient for directly observed therapy three times weekly.

    d. Discuss with the health care provider the need for the patient to use an injectable antibiotic.

4. The nurse teaches a client about the transmission of pulmonary tuberculosis (TB). Which statement made by the client indicates that teaching was effective?

    a. I will avoid being outdoors whenever possible.

    b. I will keep the windows closed at home to contain the germs.

    c. I will take the bus instead of driving to visit my friends.

    d. My husband will be sleeping in the guest bedroom.

Section VII. Asthma

Case Scenario: A 50-year-old female client is seen at the health care provider's office for a checkup. She has a history of asthma, which was more severe as a child but has improved since adolescence. She states that she exercises and does housework but gets short of breath with minimal exertion. She works as a high school principal and states her job is stressful at times. She has a negative history of smoking. She states her husband says she snores while sleeping. The client states she uses an inhaler (Ventolin) only as needed, which is when she does strenuous activities. She states she doesn't want to depend on it too much because she feels she doesn't have asthma "that bad."

Vital signs: T: 98.8, P: 82, R: 22, BP: 136/90, Weight: 196 lbs, Height: 5′3″.

Asthma

Define:

_____
_____
_____
_____

Pathophysiology/Etiology:

_____
_____
_____
_____

Risk Factors/Triggers:

_____
_____
_____
_____
_____
_____

> *Tidbit*
>
> Asthma affects millions of Americans each year. Women are more likely to have asthma than men. Over 3,000 people die from asthma each year.

Section VII. Application Exercise 1

List some of the contributing factors of asthma that this client may have.

_____
_____
_____
_____

Clinical Manifestations:

_____
_____
_____
_____

Classifications (based on severity):

Intermittent: _____

Mild: _____

Moderate: _____

Severe: _____

Diagnosis:

_____
_____
_____
_____
_____
_____
_____
_____
_____

Medication Management:

2 Classifications:

1. _____

2. _____

Medication Management (cont.)
Anti-inflammatory:

Purpose:

_____

_____
_____

Corticosteroids (action):

_____
_____
_____
_____

Names:

_____
_____
_____
_____

Leukotriene Modifiers (action):

_____
_____
_____

Names:

_____
_____
_____
_____

Anti-IgE (action):

_____
_____
_____

Names:

_____
_____
_____
_____

Medication Management (cont.)

Anti-Interleukin 5 (action):

_____
_____
_____

Names:

_____
_____
_____
_____

Bronchodilators:

Purpose:

_____
_____
_____
_____

B2-Adrengeric Agonist Drugs (action):

_____
_____
_____

Names:

SABA

_____
_____
_____
_____

LABA

_____
_____
_____
_____

Methylxanthines (action):

_____
_____
_____
_____

Names:

_____
_____
_____
_____

Anticholinergic Drugs (action):

_____
_____
_____
_____

Names:

_____
_____
_____
_____

Section VII. Application Exercise 2

Complete the table.

Inhalation Devices: As part of your client teaching, what would you instruct your patient on the use of each type of the inhalers below?

Directions for Use	Metered Dose Inhaler	Dry Powder Inhaler
Shake before use		
Inspiration		
Spacer		
Counting Device		
Inhalation per dose		
Cleaning		

Section VII. Application Exercise 3

What can you teach the client about the use of Ventolin?

_____
_____
_____
_____

Peak Flow Meter:

Purpose:

_____
_____
_____
_____
_____

How is it used?

_____
_____
_____
_____
_____

Peak Flow Zone System:

Green: _____

_____

Yellow: _____

_____

Red: _____

_____

Gerontological Considerations:

_____
_____
_____
_____
_____
_____
_____
_____
_____
_____

Section VII. Application Exercise 4

Develop 3 nursing diagnoses, goals, and interventions related to the client's status.

	Nursing Diagnosis	Goals (Client Centered)	Interventions
1.			
2.			
3.			

Match the term with the description.

1. Detailed History	Used to determine sensitivity to allergens
2. Spirometry	Used to rule out bacterial infection
3. Chest X-ray	Helps to identify asthma triggers
4. Sputum Specimen	Shows hyperinflation during an attack
5. Serum Immunoglobulin E (IgE)	Determines reversibility of bronchoconstriction and establishes diagnosis of asthma
6. Allergy Skin Test	Provides information of severity of attack and response to treatment
7. Oximetry and arterial blood gases	When elevated, highly suggests allergic tendency

Critical Thinking Questions

1. For a client with an acute asthma attack, which nursing diagnosis has the highest priority?

    a. Anxiety related to difficulty in breathing.

    b. Ineffective airway clearance related to bronchoconstriction and increased mucus production.

    c. Ineffective breathing pattern related to anxiety.

    d. Ineffective health maintenance related to lack of knowledge about attack triggers and appropriate use of medications.

2. Ineffective breathing pattern, related to decreased lung expansion during an acute attack of asthma, is an appropriate nursing diagnosis. Which nursing interventions are correct? (*Select all that apply.*)

    a. Place patient in a supine position.

    b. Administer oxygen therapy as ordered.

    c. Remain with patient during acute attack to decrease fear and anxiety.

    d. Incorporate rest periods into activities and interventions.

    e. Maintain semi-Fowler's position to facilitate ventilation.

3. The nurse teaches a patient who has asthma about peak flow meter use. Which action by the patient indicates that teaching was successful?

    a. The patient inhales rapidly through the peak flow meter mouthpiece.

    b. The patient takes montelukast (Singulair) for peak flows in the red zone.

c. The patient calls the health care provider when the peak flow is in the green zone.

d. The patient uses an albuterol (Proventil) metered dose inhaler (MDI) for peak flows in the yellow zone.

4. The emergency department nurse is evaluating the effectiveness of therapy for a patient who has received treatment during an asthma attack. Which assessment finding is the best indicator that the therapy has been effective?

a. No wheezes are audible.

b. Oxygen saturation is >90%.

c. Accessory muscle use has decreased.

d. Respiratory rate is 16 breaths/min.

Hematologic Disorders and the Disease Process of Coronary Artery Disease and Angina

Introduction

This chapter will examine hematologic disorders and the disease process of coronary artery disease and angina.

THE HEMATOLOGIC SYSTEM is made up of the blood, the spleen, bone marrow, and the liver. Hematology is the study of blood and all its components. Via the erythrocytes (red blood cells), blood carries to tissues after receiving oxygen from the respiratory system. Erythrocytes also carry away wastes. If this flow is interrupted, then all tissues will begin dying. Lack of blood flow causes myocardial infarction, strokes, and tissue death. Blood is made up of three main components: red blood cells, white blood cells, and plasma. Red blood cells, erythrocytes, are the most common blood cells. Their life span is about 100 to 120 days. **Hemoglobin (Hgb)** is the protein contained in red blood cells that is responsible for delivery of oxygen to the tissues. The **hematocrit (Hct)** measures the volume of red blood cells compared to the total blood volume (red blood cells and plasma).

Erythrocytes are filtered through the spleen. The spleen is a reservoir for blood, and it filters out erythrocytes that can no longer carry out their function. The spleen can still be removed, and the only side effects would be a slight increase in white blood cells and platelets and increased susceptibility to some diseases.

White blood cells, or leukocytes, are the body's defenders. They consist of two types: granulocytes and agranulocytes. There are six types of leukocytes. **Neutrophils** fight bacteria and fungi. **Eosinophils** fight larger parasites and modulate the inflammatory response with allergies. **Basophils** release histamine to induce an inflammatory response. There are three types of **lymphocytes:** B cells, T cells, and natural killer cells. B cells release antibodies and assist T cell activation. **T cells** can be regulatory, which cause the body to return to normal after an inflammatory response; they can activate and regulate B and T cells, or they can attack virus-infected or cancer cells. Natural killer cells attack virus-infected and tumor cells as well. **Monocytes** move to tissues and then differentiate into macrophages. **Macrophages** are phagocytic cells, and they eat cellular waste, debris, and pathogens. They also stimulate lymphocytes.

Blood is suspended in plasma. It allows blood cells to travel through the vessel of the body. Plasma, which is 90% water, allows blood cells to travel through vessels in the water it contains. Plasma is also made up of minerals, nutrients, and electrolytes. Platelets are cells that are critical to blood clotting.

The liver is responsible for cleaning the blood.

Learning Objectives of This Section

Upon completion of this chapter, the student should be able to:

- Discuss the pathophysiology and clinical manifestations of the patient with selected hematologic system alterations.
- Define terms associated with the hematologic system. Differentiate the normal and abnormal data of physical assessment of the hematologic system.
- Describe diagnostic tests for hematologic system alterations.
- Describe common hematologic system health problems.
- Describe hematologic age-related changes in the hematologic system.
- Describe the process and implement a nursing care plan to treat hematologic system alterations.
- Describe the pharmacological agents for hematologic alterations.

Section I. Anemia

Case Scenario: A resident in the skilled nursing facility is seeing the nurse in the facility's health center due to an elevated hemoglobin (Hgb) of 8.1g/dL. She is alert and oriented but is forgetful at times. She has a history of chronic obstructive pulmonary disease and congestive heart failure and kidney disease. She uses O_2 at 2 liters via nasal cannula. The resident is in the health center complaining of fatigue and shortness of breath. She states that she also has some pain in her hands due to arthritis but denies any other pain. As the nurse assesses the resident, he notes that she wears a hearing aid and dentures, along with glasses. Assessment of her lungs indicates diminished breath sounds in the bases with no adventitious sounds. She has 1+ edema bilaterally to her lower legs. She is 5′6″ tall and weighs 156 pounds.

Vital signs: T: 97.6, P: 76, R: 22, BP: 136/86, O_2 saturation is at 94%.

Self Study Guide

COMPLETE THE FOLLOWING as you listen to the lecture and/or refer to your textbook.

Anemia

Define:

_____
_____
_____
_____

Tidbit

Anemia affects an estimated 24.8% of the world's population. Preschool children have the highest risk, with an estimated 47% developing anemia globally. More than 400 types of anemia have been identified. Anemia is not restricted to humans and can affect cats and dogs.

Classifications:

Morphologic

_____
_____
_____

Etiologic

_____
_____
_____

Diagnostic Studies:

Complete Blood Count:

_____
_____
_____
_____
_____
_____

Clinical Manifestations:

_____
_____
_____
_____
_____
_____

Section I: Application Exercise 1

The resident's lab values reveal the following:

Leukocytes: 5,700 cells/mc	MCHC: 32%
RDW-CV: 15.8%	GFR: 38 mL/minute/1.73 m2
Platelets: 150,000 cells/mc	RBC: 3.02 million cells/mcL
Glucose: 82 mg/dL	Hgb: 8.1 g/dL
Blood urea nitrogen (BUN): 34 mg/dL	HCT: 25.2%
Creatinine: 1.4 mg/dL	MCV: 76 fL
MCH: 26.5 Hgb/cell	

Based on the above data, what type of anemia does the resident have based on morphology and etiology?
_____

Nursing Management:

Assessment: Subjective Data:

_____
_____
_____
_____
_____
_____
_____
_____
_____
_____
_____

Objective Data:

_____
_____
_____
_____
_____
_____
_____
_____
_____
_____

Gerontological Considerations:

_____
_____
_____
_____
_____
_____
_____
_____
_____
_____

Section I. Application Exercise 2

Due to the resident's hemoglobin levels, it is confirmed that she has anemia. She has chronic kidney disease (stage 3), which may be contributing to the anemia. Further laboratory evaluation is necessary to determine the etiology of the anemia. The health care provider orders an iron profile, vitamin B12 and folate levels, and reticulocyte count. The lab results reveal the following:

Vitamin B12: 1,996 pg/mL	Unsaturated iron binding capacity: 216 mcg/dL
Folate: 9.9 mcM	Total iron binding capacity: 452 mcg/dL
Ferritin: 11 ng/mL	Transferrin saturation: 11%
Serum iron: 26 mcg/dL	Reticulocyte count: 1%

Based on the above data, what type of anemia does the resident have? _____

Iron Deficiency Anemia

Define:

_____

_____

_____

_____

Etiology:

_____

_____

_____

_____

_____

_____

_____

_____

_____

Diagnostic Test:

_____

_____

_____

_____

_____

_____

_____

Nursing Management:

At-Risk Groups:

_____
_____
_____
_____
_____
_____
_____
_____

Medication Management:

_____
_____
_____
_____

Diet Teaching:

_____
_____
_____
_____

Megaloblastic Anemias

Cobalamin Deficiency

Define:

_____
_____
_____
_____

Etiology:

_____
_____
_____
_____
_____
_____

Clinical Manifestations:

_____
_____
_____
_____
_____
_____
_____
_____
_____
_____

Diagnostic Test:

_____
_____
_____
_____
_____
_____
_____
_____

Nursing Management:

_____
_____
_____
_____
_____
_____
_____

Folic Acid Deficiency

Define:

_____
_____
_____
_____

Etiology:

_____
_____
_____
_____

_____
_____

Clinical Manifestations:

_____
_____
_____
_____
_____
_____
_____
_____
_____
_____

Diagnostic Test:

_____
_____
_____
_____
_____
_____
_____

Nursing Management:

_____
_____
_____
_____
_____
_____
_____

Section I. Application Exercise 3

Complete the following chart.

Characteristics	Iron Deficiency Anemia	Vitamin B12 Anemia (Pernicious Anemia)	Folic Acid Deficiency
Etiology			
Clinical Manifestations			
Diagnostic Testing			
Treatment			
Food Sources			
Economic Considerations			
Food Preparation Considerations			

Critical Thinking Questions

1. When assessing a newly admitted patient, the nurse notes pallor of the skin and nail beds. The nurse should ensure that which laboratory test has been ordered?

    a. Platelet count

    b. Neutrophil count

    c. White blood cell count

    d. Hemoglobin (Hgb) level

2. What is an important teaching point for a patient who has iron deficiency anemia?

    a. Use birth control to avoid pregnancy.

    b. Increase fluids to stimulate erythropoiesis.

    c. Decrease fluid to prevent sickling of RBCs.

    d. Teaching about iron therapy medications.

3. The nurse instructs a patient about foods rich in iron. Which foods should be included in the diet?

    a. Fresh fruit and milk

    b. Cheeses and processed lunch meats

    c. Dark green leafy vegetable and organ meats

    d. Fruit juices and corn bread

4. Which statement by the patient with pernicious anemia would indicate that she understood the teaching?

    a. "I'll be glad when I can stop the injections and take only oral medicine."

    b. "I'll have to take B12 shots for the rest of my life."

    c. "After a while, I'll no longer need to take shots, just pills."

    d. "I was glad to hear that pills are available to treat me."

Section II. Coronary Artery Disease

Case Scenario: A female client, age 56, is in the clinic with complaints of chest pain that has been on and off for the last couple of days. She states that she usually walks in the evening after work but finds it difficult to do so now and has to stop and catch her breath during her walks. She says she also has some chest pain at that time. She states she smokes a pack of cigarettes a day and has been a smoker since high school. Her last visit to the physician was a couple of years ago.

Vital signs: T: 98.8, P: 70, HR: 68, R: 18.

Coronary Artery Disease

Define:

_____

_____

_____

_____

Atherosclerosis

Define:

_____

_____

_____

_____

> *Tidbit*
>
> Atherosclerosis is made up of two Greek words: *athero* ("fatty mush") and *skleros* ("hard")

Stages

1. _____

2. _____

3. _____

4. _____

Etiology/Pathophysiology

_____

_____

_____

_____

Collateral Circulation

Define:

_____

_____

_____

_____

Risk Factors

Modifiable:

_____

_____

_____
_____

Non-modifiable:

_____
_____
_____
_____

Section II. Application Exercise

What risk factors are associated with atherosclerotic plaques?

    a. Modifiable:

_____
_____

    b. Non-modifiable:

_____
_____

Nursing Management:

_____
_____
_____
_____

Gerontological Considerations:

_____
_____
_____
_____
_____
_____
_____
_____
_____
_____

Section III. Angina

Define:

_____
_____
_____
_____

Manifestations:

_____
_____
_____
_____

Diagnostic Studies

ECG

Purpose:

_____
_____
_____
_____

Cardiac Biomarkers

Purpose:

_____
_____
_____
_____

Section III. Application Exercise 1

From the previous scenario in section II:
What is likely causing Ms. Brown's angina? And what is the likely underlying cause?

_____
_____
_____
_____

Anginal Pain

Sites:

_____

_____

_____

_____

Types of Angina

Chronic Stable Angina

Prinzmetal's Angina

Define:

_____

_____

_____

_____

Acute Coronary Syndrome

Define:

_____

_____

Manifestations:

_____

_____

_____

_____

Myocardial Infarction

Define:

_____

_____

_____

_____

Healing Process:

_____
_____
_____
_____

Complications:

_____
_____
_____
_____

Section III. Application Exercise 2

What are the complications of atherosclerotic plaques along the great vessels of the body?

_____
_____
_____
_____
_____

Nursing Management:

_____
_____
_____
_____
_____
_____
_____

Stent:

_____
_____
_____
_____

Nursing Diagnosis:

_____
_____
_____
_____

Nursing Interventions/Teaching:

_____
_____
_____
_____
_____
_____
_____
_____
_____
_____
_____
_____

Critical Thinking Questions

1. A client with atherosclerosis asks a nurse which factors are responsible for this condition. What is the nurse's best response?

    a. Injury to the arteries causes them to spasm, reducing blood flow to the extremities.

    b. Excess fats in your diet are stored in the lining of your arteries, causing them to constrict.

    c. A combination of platelets and fats accumulates, narrowing the artery and reducing blood flow.

    d. Excess sodium causes injury to the arteries, reducing blood flow and eventually causing obstruction.

2. What are the following risk factors of coronary heart disease (CAD) that the nurse should discuss with a client when developing a teaching plan?

    a. Family history of coronary artery disease

    b. Increased risk associated with the patient's gender

    c. Increased risk of cardiovascular disease as people age

    d. Elevation of the patient's low-density lipoprotein (LDL) level

3. The nurse is assisting the hospitalized client with his food selections for breakfast. The client is on a low-cholesterol diet. What recommendations are most appropriate for this client?

    a. Cheese omelet, skim milk, whole wheat toast, coffee

    b. Skim milk, oatmeal, banana, orange juice, coffee

    c. Whole wheat French toast, a side of bacon, coffee

    d. Blueberry muffin, orange juice, decaffeinated coffee

4. The nurse is caring for a client with newly diagnosed hypertension. What statement by the client indicates adequate understanding of his or her diet restrictions?

    a. "I will give my canned soups to the food pantry."

    b. "I'm going to miss my evening glass of wine."

    c. "I will mostly use salt substitutes for flavoring."

    d. "I can have regular coffee only in the morning."

Use the phrases below to complete the Angina Concept Map.

1. Myocardial cells are deprived of oxygen and glucose needed for aerobic metabolism and contractility.

2. Referred cardiac pain to the shoulders, neck, lower jaw, and arms.

3. Lactic acid irritates myocardial nerve fibers and transmits a pain message to the cardiac nerves and upper thoracic posterior nerve roots.

4. Stable.

5. Atherosclerotic plaques.

6. Atypical symptoms of angina, including dyspnea, nausea, and/or fatigue.

7. Anaerobic metabolism begins and lactic acid accumulates.

8. Increased risk of MI within 3 months.

9. Variant.

10. Pain between shoulder blades.

11. Emotion.

12. Alpha receptor mediated.

13. Acute coronary syndrome.

14. Occlusion of coronary artery.

15. Vasoconstriction.

16. Exercise induced.

17. Unstable.

18. Indigestion or a burning sensation in the epigastric region.

Angina Concept Map

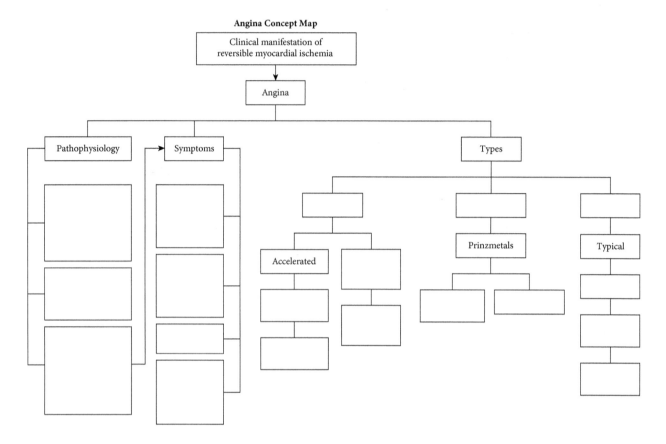

Use the word list below to complete the concept map for Medication Management.

1. Beta blocker

2. Coronary blood flow

3. Antianginal agents

4. Fixed stenosis

5. Nitrates

6. ACE inhibitors

7. Blood clot

8. Calcium channel blockers

9. Vasospasm

Concept Map Medication Management

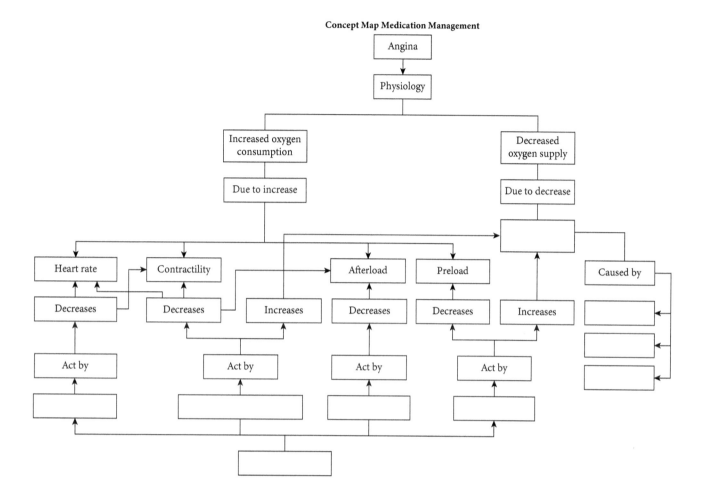

Concept Map Medication Management

Chapter 4

Perfusion Disorders and the Disease Processes Related to Perfusion

Introduction

This chapter will examine perfusion disorders and the disease processes related to perfusion.

METABOLIC PROCESSES WITHIN the cells and the body's ability to repair tissues and fight infections are dependent on perfusion and oxygenation to the tissues. During perfusion, oxygenated blood is carried to the tissues. This is done via the cardiac cycle. During systole, the heart chambers contract and blood rich in oxygen is forced into the arteries. These arteries carry blood to the tissues, and oxygen is removed. The unoxygenated blood is returned to the heart through the veins, and the cyclical process begins again after the blood is reoxygenated in the lungs. When there is an interruption in this process, the body is not receiving adequate circulation and disease develops.

Learning Objectives of This Section

Upon completion of this chapter, the student should be able to:

- Discuss the pathophysiology and clinical manifestations of cardiac perfusion problems.
- Define terms associated with the cardiac perfusion system.
- Differentiate the normal and abnormal data of physical assessment of the cardiac perfusion system.
- Describe diagnostic tests for cardiac perfusion system alterations.
- Describe common cardiac perfusion health problems.
- Describe age-related changes in cardiac perfusion systems.
- Describe the process and implement a nursing care plan to treat cardiac perfusion system alterations.
- Describe the pharmacological agents for cardiac system alterations.

Section I. Peripheral Vascular Disease

Case Scenario: A 68-year-old client is being admitted to the unit after a visit to the health care provider's office. He is complaining of pain in lower extremities when ambulating. He has a history of hypertension and takes care of himself. As you begin to examine the client, you notice that he has a bandage on his right foot that he says he keeps on so that his shoes don't rub on his foot.

Peripheral Artery Disease

Define:

_____
_____
_____
_____

Etiology/Pathophysiology:

_____
_____
_____
_____

Arteries Affected:

_____
_____
_____
_____

Manifestations:

_____
_____
_____
_____

Complications:

_____
_____
_____
_____

Diagnostic Studies:

_____
_____
_____
_____

Section I. Application Exercise 1

As you admit the client onto the unit and his room, prioritize the nursing interventions you would do for the client. Write the number in the box and list your rationale for each intervention.

Interventions	Number of Priority	Rationale
Take vital signs		
Assess bilateral pedal pulses		
Orient client to room		
Conduct health assessment		
Apply sterile dressing to right foot		

Nursing Diagnosis:

_____
_____
_____
_____

Planning:

_____
_____
_____
_____

Nursing Implementation/Management:

_____
_____
_____
_____
_____
_____
_____
_____

Evaluation:

_____
_____
_____
_____

Section I. Application Exercise 2

As you assess the client, you notice that he is alert and oriented. He is ambulatory and as he returns to bed from the bathroom, you assess that he has a reddish-blue color to bilateral lower extremities, 1+ edema, and both of the extremities are cool to the touch. Thready pulses are also noted bilaterally.

Determine two nursing diagnoses for the client and what your interventions would be for these diagnoses. Include rationale.

Nursing Diagnosis	Nursing Interventions	Rationale

Section II. Venous Thromboembolism/Venous and Arterial Insufficiency

Case Scenario: A 50-year-old female presents to the health care provider's office complaining of pain in her right calf. She states that she had appendicitis surgery 3 weeks ago, and the pain in her right calf started a week ago. She states the pain in her calf has progressed to her right thigh. As you gather data on her health history, you note that she did not receive any blood thinners while she was in the hospital. Your assessment findings are:

- T: 98.8, P: 72, R: 16, BP: 126/70.
- Right leg is swollen and measurements are: left calf 36 cm, left thigh 30 cm, right calf 54 cm, right thigh 51cm. Her medical records do not indicate that she received VTE prophylaxis while in hospital. She has no significant past medical history.

Venous Thromboembolism

Define:

Thrombus

_____

_____

Phlebitis

_____

_____

Thrombophlebitis

_____

_____

Pulmonary Embolism

_____

_____

Virchow's Triad

_____

_____

_____

> **Tidbit**
>
> Venous thromboembolism (VTE) is a process that includes pulmonary embolism (PE) and deep vein thrombosis (DVT).

Management:

_____

_____

Section II. Application Exercise 1

You suspect that a client has a deep vein thrombosis. What would you do next?

_____

_____

_____

_____

_____

Venous Insufficiency

Define:

_____

_____

_____

_____

Treatment:

_____

_____

_____

_____

Arterial Insufficiency

Define:

_____

_____

_____

_____

Treatment:

_____

_____

_____

_____

Tidbit

Venous ulcers result from venous insufficiency. They typically occur on the malleolus (ankle) or the medial aspect of the leg superior to the malleolus. The ulcer is shallow, irregular, ruddy, and granulating. The client may have aching leg pain when legs are dependent because of edema, or there may be no pain associated with the ulcer unless superficial nerves are exposed.

Tidbit

Arterial insufficiency is most often due to atherosclerosis. In atherosclerosis, the arteries become narrowed from deposits of fatty substances in the arterial vessel walls, often due to high levels of cholesterol and aggravated by smoking and high blood pressure (hypertension). The arteries fail to deliver oxygen and nutrients to the leg and foot, resulting in tissue breakdown.

Section II. Application Exercise 2

Complete the table.

Signs and Symptoms	Arterial Disorder	Venous Disorder
Pain		
Pulses		
Edema		
Skin Changes		

Critical Thinking Questions

1. What symptom would indicate possible thrombophlebitis?

   a. Pain along a vein

   b. Severe cramping

   c. Edema

   d. Area around a vein that is warm to the touch

2. Which topic should the nurse include in patient teaching for a patient with a venous stasis ulcer on the left lower leg?

   a. Need to increase carbohydrate intake

   b. Methods of keeping the wound area dry

   c. Purpose of prophylactic antibiotic therapy

   d. Application of elastic compression stockings

3. The nurse assesses a client's legs. Which assessment finding indicates arterial insufficiency?

   a. Ankle discoloration and pitting edema

   b. Dependent mottling and absence of hair

   c. Pain with activity but not while resting

   d. Full veins present in dependent extremity

4. Which patient statement to the nurse is most consistent with the diagnosis of venous insufficiency?

   a. "I can't get my shoes on at the end of the day."

   b. "I can't ever seem to get my feet warm enough."

   c. "I have burning leg pains after I walk two blocks."

   d. "I wake up during the night because my legs hurt."

Chapter 5

Cardiac Alterations—Perfusion

Introduction

This chapter will examine specific cardiac perfusion disorders and the disease processes related to cardiac perfusion.

A NY ALTERATION IN cardiac perfusion causes problems with oxygenation to the heart and vital organs. Underlying mechanisms or causative factors will depend on the disease process that is involved and thus display various symptoms. The inability for the heart to supply sufficient blood to the body's tissue to meet metabolic demand results in cerebrovascular disease and heart failure.

Learning Objectives of This Section

Upon completion of this chapter, the student should be able to:

- Discuss the pathophysiology and clinical manifestations of cardiac perfusion problems.
- Define terms associated with the cardiac perfusion system.
- Differentiate the normal and abnormal data of physical assessment of the cardiac perfusion system.
- Describe diagnostic tests for cardiac perfusion system alterations.
- Describe common cardiac perfusion health problems.
- Describe age-related changes in cardiac perfusion systems.
- Describe the process and implement a nursing care plan to treat cardiac perfusion system alterations.
- Describe the pharmacological agents for cardiac perfusion system alterations.
- Demonstrate safe performance of skills used in caring for individuals with cardiac perfusion problems.

Section I. Myocardial Infarction

Case Scenario: A 52-year-old client presents to the emergency department with complaints of chest pain, which he describes as a "heaviness" in his mid-chest with pain radiating to his back, neck, and down his left arm. He rates his pain as a 5 out of 10. The client states he has been a smoker and has a family history of cardiovascular disease. The client has a positive history for hypertension, for which he states he takes Vasotec daily. He is 5'6" tall and weighs 256 lbs. The client is placed on a cardiac monitor and has his cardiac enzymes drawn. The monitor shows ST elevation, T inversion, and pathologic Q wave. His cardiac enzyme CK is elevated along with his LDH and AST elevations. He has been diagnosed with myocardial infarction (MI).

Vital signs: T: 98.8, P: 100, R: 22, BP: 160/96.

Self Study Guide
COMPLETE THE FOLLOWING as you listen to the lecture and/or refer to your textbook.

Myocardial Infarction

Define:

_____
_____
_____
_____

Healing Process:

_____
_____
_____
_____

Complications:

_____
_____
_____
_____

> ### Tidbit
> Myocardial infarction is part of the group of disorders called acute coronary syndrome.

Section I. Application Exercise 1
What risk factors for myocardial infarction (MI) is the client presenting in the above scenario? What are some other assessment data that the nurse should collect related to cardiovascular disease?

Risk Factors:

_____
_____

Other Assessment Data:

_____
_____
_____

Nursing Management:

_____
_____
_____
_____
_____
_____
_____
_____
_____

Stent:

_____
_____
_____
_____

Nursing Diagnosis:

_____
_____
_____
_____

Nursing Interventions/Teaching:

_____
_____
_____
_____
_____
_____
_____
_____
_____
_____

Section I. Application Exercise 2

The client continues to complain of chest pain and is given IV nitroglycerin (NTG) and is on 2 liters of O_2 via nasal cannula.

What can the continued chest pain indicate, and how do NTG and oxygen play a role in controlling pain in MI clients?

Continued pain indicates?

_____
_____
_____
_____

Role of NTG and oxygen with controlling pain.

_____
_____
_____
_____

Section I. Application Exercise 3

The client's pain has been under control, and there have been no further dysrhythmias noted. The nurse is preparing the client and his wife for discharge.

His discharge instructions include:

- 2gm Na, low fat, low cholesterol
- Begin cardiac rehab tomorrow
- Follow-up with health care provider within a week
- Medications: Continue Vasotec at 5mg daily

  o Aspirin 81mg daily
  o Colace 100mg daily

How can the nurse assess if the client and his wife understand the discharge instructions?

_____
_____
_____
_____
_____
_____
_____
_____
_____
_____
_____

Section II. Heart Failure

Case Scenario: Mrs. C., 74 years old, is your client on the unit today. She has 3+ pitting edema to bilateral lower extremities and is complaining of shortness of breath (SOB). Her respirations are 30, and she has a cough producing frothy, blood-tinged sputum. She states she cannot remember if she ate her breakfast or had her medications this morning. You have given her medications to her earlier with her breakfast. She has a diagnosis of congestive heart failure.

Vital signs: T: 98, P: 70, R: 30, BP: 176/100.

Orders include: Q 4hr vital signs, up in chair QID, O_2 at 2l nasal cannula, Foley catheter, I&O

Diet: Low Na+, soft

Labs: serum K+, ABGs, ECG, Chest X-ray

IV D5W at 50mL/hr

Heart Failure

Define:

_____

_____

_____

_____

> *Tidbit*
>
> Heart failure is increasing in prevalence due to improved survival after cardiovascular events and increased population of older adults.

Etiology/Pathophysiology:

_____

_____

_____

_____

_____

_____

_____

_____

_____

Section II. Application Exercise 1

Place an "X" in the corresponding box to determine which is a sign or symptom of left-sided or right-sided heart failure.

		Left-sided Failure	Right-sided Failure
Signs	• Murmurs • Alternating pulses, strong, weak • Jugular vein distention • Changes in mental status • Hepatomegaly • Ascites • Crackles • Increased heart rate • Weight gain • S3 & S4 heart sounds • Restlessness, confusion • Anasarca • Poor O_2 exchange		
Symptoms	• Fatigue • Nocturia • Anxiety, depression • Dry, hacking cough • Frothy, pink-tinged sputum • Nausea • Dyspnea • Right upper-quadrant pain • Shallow, rapid respirations • Anorexia, GI bloating • Dependent bilateral edema • Paroxysmal nocturnal dyspnea • Orthopnea		

Cardiac Biomarkers

Define:

_____
_____
_____
_____

Troponin T

Define:

_____
_____

Rises _____

Peaks _____

How long is it detected? _____

Troponin I

Define:

_____

_____

Rises _____

Peaks _____

How long is it detected? _____

Creatine Kinase (CK)

Define:

_____

Creatine Kinase MB (CK-MB)

Define:

_____

_____

Rises _____

Peaks _____

How long is it detected?

_____

Copeptin

Define:

_____

_____

Myoglobin

Define:

_____
_____
_____

Blood Studies

B-type Natriuretic Peptides (BNP)

Define:

_____
_____

Homocysteine

Define:

_____
_____

C-Reactive Protein

Define:

_____
_____

Serum Lipids

Triglycerides

Define:

_____
_____

Cholesterol

Define:

_____
_____

Phospholipids

Define:

_____

_____

Lipoproteins

Chylomicrons

Define:

_____

_____

Low-density Lipoproteins

Define:

_____

_____

Very Low-density Lipoproteins

Define:

_____

_____

High-density Lipoproteins

Define:

_____

_____

Diagnostic Assessment

Electrocardiogram

Define:

_____

_____

Echocardiogram

Define:

_____
_____

Transesophageal Echocardiogram

Define:

_____
_____

Stress Electrocardiogram

Define:

_____
_____

Cardiac Catheterization

Define:

_____
_____
_____
_____
_____
_____
_____
_____
_____
_____

Care of the patient with cardiac catheterization

_____
_____
_____
_____
_____
_____

Cardiac Output

Define:

_____
_____

Preload

Define:

_____
_____

Afterload

Define:

_____
_____

Contractility

Define:

_____
_____

Medical Management:

_____
_____
_____
_____
_____
_____
_____
_____
_____

Section II. Application Exercise 2

Look at the nursing interventions for the client below and put them in priority order. Then, next to each, write your evidence-based rationale for each intervention.

_____   *Check current lab data*   _____

_____

_____

_____

_____   *Assess respiratory rate*   _____

_____

_____

_____   *Assess rate/rhythm, quality of pulse*   _____

_____

_____

_____

_____   *Obtain I&O*   _____

_____

_____

_____

Nursing Management

Assessment:

_____
_____
_____
_____
_____
_____
_____

Diagnosis:

_____
_____
_____
_____

Planning:

_____
_____
_____
_____
_____
_____
_____
_____
_____

Interventions:

_____
_____
_____
_____
_____
_____
_____
_____

Evaluation:

_____
_____
_____
_____
_____
_____
_____
_____

Gerontological Considerations with Cardiovascular Disease

_____
_____
_____
_____
_____

_____

_____

_____

_____

_____

_____

_____

_____

_____

Section II. Application Exercise 3

You are in Mrs. C.'s room to provide hygiene care for her. You assess the following: 2+ lower extremity edema, respirations 22 and crackles heard bilaterally, skin cool to the touch. Mrs. C. is alert and oriented but states she is weak and needs help with her bath.

Using the nursing diagnoses below, prioritize each diagnosis. List your interventions and the rationale for each.

Nursing Diagnoses:

- *Excess fluid volume, anxiety*
- *Fatigue, impaired tissue integrity*
- *Activity intolerance*
- *Risk for injury, knowledge deficit*
- *Impaired gas exchange.*

Nursing Diagnosis	Rationale	Nursing Interventions

Section III. Cerebrovascular Accident (CVA)

Case Scenario: A 60-year-old male client is seen in the emergency department with right-sided weakness, expressive aphasia, and homonymous hemianopia. He is lethargic, and his history reveals a 20-year smoking habit and he has abused drugs and alcohol in the past. His wife is with him and states he began complaining of not being able to pick up his fork to eat and seemed very drowsy. He is 6 ft tall and weighs 250 lbs.

Vital signs: T: 98.8, P: 94, R: 22, BP: 190/110.

Stroke

Define:

_____
_____
_____
_____

Tidbit

The terms brain attack and cerebrovascular accident are also used to describe stroke. It is the fifth most common cause of death in the United States.

Classification:

1. _____

    a. _____

    b. _____

2. _____

TIA:

Define: _____

_____
_____
_____
_____

Section III. Application Exercise 1

Describe the terms *expressive aphasia* and *homonymous hemianopia* and the nursing responsibilities for each.

Expressive Aphasia: Definition	Nursing Care
Homonymous Hemianopias: Definition	Nursing Care

Warning Signs of a Stroke: FAST acronym

F: _____

A: _____

S: _____

T: _____

Manifestations:

Left-Side Stroke	Right-Side Stroke

Section III. Application Exercise 2

Looking at the above case scenario, what are the risk factors and how might they cause a CVA?
Risk Factors:

_____
_____
_____
_____
_____
_____

Risk Factors:

Modifiable: Define and List

_____
_____
_____
_____

Non-modifiable: Define and List

_____
_____
_____
_____

Section III. Application Exercise 3

The client is scheduled for a CT scan and cerebral angiogram. His tests reveal that he has a blockage in his mid-cerebral artery. It is definitive that he has had a CVA. What nursing diagnoses are appropriate for the client at this time?

1. _____
2. _____
3. _____
4. _____
5. _____
6. _____

Diagnostic Tests:

_____
_____

_____
_____
_____
_____
_____
_____
_____
_____
_____

Nursing Management:

Subjective Data:

_____
_____
_____
_____
_____

Objective Data:

_____
_____
_____
_____
_____

Neurological Exam:

_____
_____
_____
_____
_____

Nursing Interventions Related to Each System

Respiratory:

_____
_____
_____
_____
_____

Cardiovascular:

_____
_____
_____
_____
_____
_____

Musculoskeletal:

_____
_____
_____
_____
_____
_____

Integumentary:

_____
_____
_____
_____
_____
_____

Gastrointestinal:

_____
_____
_____
_____
_____
_____

Urinary:

_____
_____
_____
_____
_____

Nutrition:

_____
_____
_____
_____
_____
_____

Communication:

_____
_____
_____
_____
_____
_____

Sensory:

_____
_____
_____
_____
_____
_____

Psychosocial:

_____
_____
_____
_____
_____
_____

Gerontological Considerations:

_____
_____
_____
_____
_____
_____
_____
_____

_____

_____

_____

_____

Critical Thinking Questions

1. A patient is admitted to the hospital with a diagnosis of transient ischemic attack (TIA). The patient asks the nurse to explain to him what a TIA is. Which statement by the nurse is most accurate?

   a. A TIA is a result of permanent cerebrovascular insufficiency.

   b. An episode of a TIA may last up to 2 days.

   c. A TIA is often a precursor to a stroke.

   d. A TIA generally occurs once and never occurs again.

2. A right-handed patient has right-sided hemiplegia and aphasia from a stroke. Where is the most likely location of the lesion?

   a. Left frontal lobe

   b. Right brainstem

   c. Motor areas of the right cerebrum

   d. Medial superior area of the temporal lobe

3. A patient experiencing TIAs is scheduled for a carotid endarterectomy. The patient asks the nurse what this procedure is. The nurse gives which response?

   a. This procedure promotes cerebral flow to decrease cerebral edema.

   b. This procedure reduces the brain damage that occurs during a stroke.

   c. This procedure helps prevent a stroke by removing atherosclerotic plaques obstructing cerebral blood flow.

   d. This procedure provides a circulatory bypass around thrombotic plaques obstructing cranial circulation.

4. What nursing interventions should the nurse include in the plan of care for a client who has had a stroke with right-sided hemiplegia and expressive aphasia? (*Select all that apply.*)

   a. Allow the patient ample time to verbalize his needs.

   b. Encourage self-help behaviors as much as possible, such as feeding.

   c. Monitor the patient's neurologic status once a day.

   d. Perform ROM to affected extremities every shift.

   e. Implement the use of a communication board for the patient to use as needed.

5. The nurse is assessing the client with congestive heart failure. The client is restless and has crackles and wheezes in the lower bases and respirations are 26. What is the priority intervention at this time?

   a. Assess fluid intake

   b. Keep client in bed

   c. Check pulse oximetry

   d. Assess capillary refill

6. The client with heart failure is put on O_2 at 2 liters via nasal cannula. The client asks why he has to use oxygen. What is the nurse's best response? (*Select all that apply.*)

   a. O_2 assists with meeting tissue oxygen needs.

   b. It helps relieve dyspnea and fatigue.

   c. It will help during aerobic exercise.

   d. It improves oxygen saturation.

7. The heart failure client is on a low-sodium diet. What should be removed from her tray by the nurse?

   a. Tomato soup

   b. Fresh mixed vegetables

   c. Broiled fish

   d. Dinner roll

8. The heart failure client is being discharged. What statement indicates that teaching has been effective for activity? (*Select all that apply.*)

   a. "I will avoid extremes of heat and cold."

   b. "I will increase walking gradually as long as it does not cause fatigue or shortness of breath."

   c. "I can exercise to the point of exertion."

   d. "It is important to plan a regular rest and activity program."

Chapter 6

Upper Gastrointestinal Alterations

Introduction

This chapter will examine upper gastrointestinal alterations and the disease processes related to them.

THE GASTROINTESTINAL (GI) tract consists of organs that extend from the mouth to the anus. These organs are hollow and are a part of the digestive system. Organs in the GI tract are the mouth, esophagus, stomach, small and large intestines, and the anus. These organs, along with the liver, pancreas, and gallbladder, help to take in food and nutrients and aid in the digestive process. Blood vessels also help in transporting nutrients to other parts of the body. In the digestive system, the role of the nervous system and hormones is to regulate the function of the GI flora to control immunity, digestion, and maintain homeostasis. There are several different diseases that can affect the GI tract and impact the individual's overall health status.

Learning Objectives of This Chapter

Upon completion of this chapter, the student should be able to:

- Discuss the pathophysiology and clinical manifestations of upper gastrointestinal problems.
- Describe age-related changes in the upper gastrointestinal system.
- Describe common upper gastrointestinal health problems.
- Describe the nursing process in which upper gastrointestinal problems may occur.
- Identify common upper gastrointestinal medications.
- Identify important components of a subjective and objective upper gastrointestinal health history.

Section I. Nausea and Vomiting

Case Scenario: A 46-year-old male presents to the emergency department with a two-day history of vomiting. The client is accompanied by his wife. The client states that when he tries to eat, he becomes very nauseous. His wife states that this has occurred with each meal. He denies abdominal pain, diarrhea, or constipation. The client also states that he tried milk of magnesia, but it has not helped.

Vital signs: T: 98.8, P: 96, R: 20, BP: 146/92.

Self Study Guide

COMPLETE THE FOLLOWING as you listen to the lecture and/or refer to your textbook.

Nausea and Vomiting

Define:

_____
_____
_____
_____

Etiology/Pathophysiology:

_____
_____
_____
_____

Manifestations:

_____
_____
_____
_____

Complications:

_____
_____
_____
_____

Tidbit
Nausea and vomiting are the most common manifestations of GI diseases. Although each manifestation can occur independently, they are closely related and treated as one problem.

Section I. Application Exercise 1

The client was seen by the physician and received the following orders:

- NPO
- IV fluids of 0.9% NaCl at 50ml/hr
- Strict I&O
- NG to low intermittent suction
- Reglan 5 mg IV q 6 hrs

Develop a nursing care plan related to the client's signs and symptoms.

Nursing Diagnosis	Client Goals	Interventions	Rationale

Section II. Gastroesophageal Reflux Disease

Define:

_____

_____

_____

_____

Tidbit

About 10–20% of the U.S. population experience GERD symptoms at least once a week.

Section II. Application Exercise 1

After 24 hours, the client's symptoms have subsided, and the NG tube was removed. The patient began on a clear liquid diet with advanced as tolerated. The client reveals to the health care provider that before he began experiencing the nausea and vomiting episodes, he was having heartburn for several weeks. The health care provider ordered an endoscopy, and it was revealed that the client has gastroesophageal reflux disease. The wife asks, "How this could happen? I don't cook a lot of greasy foods."

   Explain to the client and his wife the cause of GERD.

Etiology/Pathophysiology:

_____
_____
_____
_____
_____
_____
_____
_____
_____
_____
_____

Manifestations:

_____
_____
_____
_____
_____
_____
_____
_____
_____

Section II. Application Exercise 2

List the medications related to GERD.

Medications

Histamine Receptor Blockers Action:	Proton Pump Inhibitors Action:	Prokinetic Agents Action:

Complications

Barrett's Esophagus:

_____
_____
_____

Esophagitis:

_____
_____
_____
_____

Diagnostic Studies:

_____
_____
_____
_____
_____
_____
_____
_____
_____
_____

Collaborative Care

Surgery

Nissen Fundoplication

_____
_____
_____
_____

LINX

_____
_____
_____
_____

Endoscopic Therapy

_____
_____
_____
_____

Nursing Management

Assessment:

_____
_____
_____
_____

Diagnosis:

_____
_____
_____
_____

Planning/Interventions:

_____
_____
_____
_____

Evaluation:

_____
_____
_____
_____

Postoperative Care:

_____
_____
_____
_____
_____
_____
_____

Section II. Application Exercise 3

After treatment for GERD, the client is being sent home. The nurse has been assigned to develop a teaching plan for the client. List what the nurse should include in her teaching plan for the client and his wife. Are there any other health care professionals that should be included in the teaching plan?

Client and Caregiver Teaching Plan

1. _____   6. _____

2. _____   7. _____

3. _____   8. _____

4. _____   9. _____

5. _____   10. _____

Section III. Gastritis

Case Scenario: The nurse is assigned to care for a client on the unit who has been admitted with complaints of feeling full and having episodes of nausea and vomiting. The patient has a history of chronic back pain and alcohol abuse. He states he takes ibuprofen daily to manage the pain.

> *Tidbit*
>
> Gastritis is one of the most common problems affecting the stomach.

Define:

_____
_____
_____
_____

Etiology/Pathophysiology:

_____
_____
_____
_____

Helicobacter pylori (*H. pylori*)

Define:

_____
_____

Section III. Application Exercise 1

The client is diagnosed with gastritis. Match the type of gastritis to the definition.

Types

Acute gastritis	Inflammation and wearing down of the stomach lining
Chronic gastritis	Changes in the stomach lining
Erosive gastritis	Associated with alcohol abuse; lasts for a few hours to days
Non-erosive gastritis	Causes pernicious anemia and neurologic complications

Manifestations:

_____
_____
_____
_____

Diagnostic Studies:

_____
_____
_____
_____
_____
_____
_____
_____

Medical Management:

_____
_____
_____
_____
_____
_____
_____

Nursing Management

Assessment:

_____
_____
_____

_____

_____

_____

_____

Diagnosis:

_____

_____

_____

_____

Planning/Interventions:

_____

_____

_____

_____

_____

_____

_____

_____

Evaluation:

_____

_____

_____

_____

_____

_____

_____

_____

Section IV. Peptic Ulcer Disease

Case Scenario: A 45-year-old woman is in the health care provider's office complaining of "stomachaches." She states that the pain occurs several times a day, usually between meals. She rates the pain a 4 out of 10 and states that the pain is like a burning, achy pain. The client states that eating makes the pain go away, but it returns a few hours later. She has taken over-the-counter antacids. The doctor has ordered an endoscopy.

Define:

_____

_____

> _Tidbit_
>
> In the United States, peptic ulcer disease (PUD) affects approximately 4.5 million people annually. Approximately 10% of the U.S. population has evidence of a duodenal ulcer at some time.

_____
_____

Types

Acute:

_____
_____
_____
_____

Chronic:

_____
_____
_____
_____

Etiology/Pathophysiology:

_____
_____
_____
_____
_____
_____
_____
_____

Manifestations:

_____
_____
_____
_____

Diagnostic Tests:

_____
_____
_____
_____

Section IV. Application Exercise 1

The endoscopy results indicate that the client has a peptic ulcer and the presence of *Helicobacter pylori* (*H. pylori*) is seen. Gastric and duodenal ulcers are types of peptic ulcers.

Use the chart below to compare the differences between gastric and duodenal ulcers.

Characteristics	Gastric	Duodenal
Lesion		
Location of Lesion		
Gastric Secretion		
Incidence		
Clinical Manifestations		
Recurrence Rate		

Medication Management

Antacids:

_____

_____

_____

_____

Histamine (H2) Receptor Blockers:

_____

_____

_____

_____

Proton Pump Inhibitors:

_____

_____

_____

_____

Mucosal Healing Agent:

_____

_____

_____

_____

Antisecretory and Cytoprotective Agent:

_____

_____

_____

_____

Section IV. Application Exercise 2

The client has been placed on antibiotics to treat the *H. pylori* infection for 10 days and omeprazole for the hyperacidity. Develop a teaching plan for the client in managing his peptic ulcer.

Dietary management
Cigarette smoking
Alcohol intake

Medication management
Stress management
Lifestyle changes

Nursing Management

Assessment:

_____
_____
_____
_____
_____

Diagnosis:

_____
_____
_____
_____

Planning/Implementation:

_____
_____
_____
_____
_____
_____
_____

Evaluation:

_____

_____

_____

_____

Section V. Gallbladder Disease

Case Scenario: A 38-year-old male presents to the emergency department complaining of abdominal pain, nausea, and vomiting. He states he has had abdominal pain before, but it has gone away. He states that the pain today will not go away, and on a scale of 1–10, the pain is at an 8, and he states it is like a dull, cramping pain. The client is grabbing his abdomen and appears very uncomfortable. The location of the pain is in the right upper quadrant, and the client says it radiates to his back. History includes hypertension.

Vital signs: T: 100.2, P: 110, R: 20, BP: 150/94, Ht: 5'5″, Wt: 256 lbs.

Tidbit

The incidence of gallbladder disease is a common problem in the United States. Cholelithiasis is higher in women over the age of 40, postmenopausal women, and young women on contraceptives.

Cholelithiasis

Define:

_____

_____

_____

Cholecystitis

Define:

_____

_____

_____

Risk Factors:

_____

_____

_____

Etiology/Pathophysiology:

_____

_____

_____

_____

_____

_____

_____

Manifestations:

_____

_____

_____

_____

Complications:

_____

_____

_____

_____

Section V. Application Exercise 1

The health care provider has ordered the following diagnostic studies. Fill in the chart below on the diagnostic tests for the patient.

Test	Purpose
Ultrasound	
Endoscopic retrograde cholangiopancreatography (ERCP)	
Percutaneous transhepatic cholangiography	
Liver Enzymes	
Pancreatic Enzymes	

WBC	
Direct Bilirubin	
Indirect Bilirubin	

Medical Management:

_____

_____

_____

_____

Lithotripsy:

_____

_____

_____

_____

Cholecystectomy:

_____

_____

_____

_____

Section V. Application Exercise2

The test results for the client reveal an elevated WBC count, liver enzymes elevated, and the ERCP and ultrasound show a stone in the common bile duct. The client has been diagnosed with acute cholecystitis and has been scheduled for laparoscopic cholecystectomy. Develop a postoperative teaching plan for the client.

Postoperative Instructions	Instructions to Client
Wound care	
Signs and symptoms to notify health care provider	
Activity	
Diet	

Nursing Management

Assessment:

_____
_____
_____
_____

Diagnosis:

_____
_____
_____
_____

Planning/Interventions:

_____
_____
_____
_____

Evaluation:

_____
_____
_____
_____

Section VI. Hiatal Hernia

Case Scenario: A client presents to the immediate care center with complaints of heartburn and chest and abdominal pain. She states that she has some shortness of breath and has had dark stools and vomiting. The health care provider schedules an upper endoscopy.

Hiatal Hernia

Define:

_____
_____
_____
_____

Types

Sliding:

_____
_____
_____

Rolling or Paraesophageal:

_____
_____
_____

Diagnostic Studies:

_____
_____
_____
_____

Medical Management:

_____
_____
_____
_____
_____
_____
_____
_____

Section VI. Application Exercise 1

The endoscopy shows that the client has a sliding hiatal hernia. The health care provider has ordered a proton pump inhibitor (PPI). Develop a drug card for proton pump inhibitors that you can use to teach the client about the drug.

Drug Card

Proton Pump Inhibitor (PPI) purpose: _____

Name brands for PPIs: _____

Side Effects: _____

Nursing Management

Assessment:

_____
_____
_____
_____

Diagnosis:

_____
_____
_____
_____

Planning/Implementation:

_____
_____
_____
_____
_____
_____
_____

Evaluation:

_____
_____
_____
_____

Critical Thinking Questions

1. A 35-year-old man has been admitted with a diagnosis of peptic ulcers. Which drugs would the nurse expect to be prescribed for him to decrease gastric acid secretion?

   a. Maalox and Kayexalate

   b. Tagamet and Zantac

   c. Erythromycin and Flagyl

   d. Dyazide and Carafate

2. The 92-year-old client is dehydrated from diarrhea, exhibits anorexia and has lost 1 lb since yesterday. To help stimulate intake, the nurse would: (*Select all that apply.*)

   a. Moisten the patient's mouth with mouthwash.

   b. Put away bedpans and urinals.

   c. Leave the patient in privacy during mealtime.

   d. Check the fit of the patient's dentures.

   e. Offer favorite food.

3. Which item should the nurse offer to the patient who is to restart oral intake after being NPO due to nausea and vomiting?

   a. Glass of grape juice

   b. Dish of orange gelatin

   c. Cup of hot chocolate

   d. Bowl of hot chicken broth

4. A 42-year-old male with gastroesophageal reflux disease (GERD) is experiencing increasing discomfort. Which patient statement indicates that additional teaching about GERD is needed?

   a. "I take antacids between meals and at bedtime each night."

   b. "I sleep with the head of the bed elevated on 4-inch blocks."

   c. "I eat small meals during the day and have a bedtime snack."

   d. "I quit smoking several years ago, but I still chew a lot of gum."

Chapter 7

Lower Gastrointestinal Alterations

Introduction

This chapter will examine lower gastrointestinal alterations and the disease processes related to them.

T HE GASTROINTESTINAL (GI) tract consists of organs that extend from the mouth to the anus. These organs are hollow and are a part of the digestive system. Organs in the GI tract are the mouth, esophagus, stomach, small and large intestines, and the anus. These organs, along with the liver, pancreas, and gallbladder, help to take in food and nutrients and aid in the digestive process. Blood vessels also help in transporting nutrients to other parts of the body. The role of the nervous system and hormones in the digestive system is to regulate the function of the GI flora to control immunity, digestion, and maintain homeostasis. There are several different diseases that can affect the GI tract and impact the individual's overall health status.

Learning Objectives of This Chapter

Upon completion of this chapter, the student should be able to:

- Discuss the pathophysiology and clinical manifestations of lower gastrointestinal problems.
- Describe age-related changes in the lower gastrointestinal system.
- Describe common lower gastrointestinal health problems.
- Describe the nursing process in which lower gastrointestinal problems may occur.
- Identify common lower gastrointestinal medications.
- Identify important components of a subjective and objective lower gastrointestinal health history.

Section I. Appendicitis

Case Scenario: A 28-year-old female presents at the emergency department with complaints of abdominal pain. She is accompanied by her mother. The client states the pain began as a dull pain in the "center of my stomach, right at the belly button" and has now moved to the right side. She states the pain is worse when she moves and is persistent. She rates it as an 8 out of 10 on the pain scale. The client's mother states that the client has also had some nausea and vomiting. Nursing assessment reveals:

Vitals: T: 100.3, P: 90, R: 28, BP: 130/88.

Localized and rebound tenderness with the client displaying a guarding position with right leg flexed.

Self Study Guide

COMPLETE THE FOLLOWING as you listen to the lecture and/or refer to your textbook.

Appendicitis

Define:

_____
_____
_____
_____

Etiology/Pathophysiology:

_____
_____
_____
_____
_____

McBurney's Point:

_____
_____
_____

Manifestations:

_____
_____
_____
_____

Section I. Application Exercise 1

The client was seen by the physician and received the following orders:

- NPO
- IV fluids of 0.9% NS @100ml/hr
- CBC ordered
- Urinalysis
- CT scan and ultrasound

- Surgical consult
- Strict I&O

The following diagnosis applies to this patient:

Fluid volume deficit, knowledge deficit, anxiety, pain, activity intolerance, self-care deficit.

Determine a priority diagnosis and write client outcome, interventions, and rationale for the diagnosis.

Nursing Diagnosis	Client Outcome	Interventions	Rationale

Diagnostic Tests:

_____
_____
_____
_____

Nursing Management (Preoperatively):

_____
_____
_____
_____
_____
_____
_____
_____

Section I. Application Exercise 2

The client has been diagnosed with acute appendicitis. The client has been scheduled for an appendectomy. The client is prepared for surgery and has the procedure via laparoscopy. The appendix was not ruptured, so there were no complications with the surgery. Client is taken to the PACU for postoperative assessment. She has a dressing to her right lower quadrant. The client remains stable and is transferred to the unit.

You are the nurse on the unit assigned to care for the client. Implement a teaching plan for the client, including discharge instructions.

Teaching Plan

Activity	Medications	Wound Care

Section II. Irritable Bowel Disease

Case Scenario: Mrs. Thompson, a 38-year-old single mother of two boys, is seen in the health care provider's office today. She states that she has had bouts of stomach pain and feeling bloated for the last few days, especially after eating. The client states she also has had some loose stools alternating with constipation, in which the pain subsides a bit after a bowel movement. She states she has been stressed due to her job as a bus driver and taking care of her sons. The client states she has a history of GERD.

Nursing assessment reveals:

Vitals: T: 99.0, P: 88, R: 24, BP: 148/90. Skin warm and dry. Lungs clear, no peripheral edema. Hyperactive bowel sounds in left lower quadrant.

Tidbit

IBS is more frequently diagnosed in women than in men.

Irritable Bowel Disease

Define:

_____
_____
_____
_____

Etiology/Pathophysiology:

Types

1. _____

2. _____

3. _____

Section II. Application Exercise 1

The physician has ordered a CT scan, sigmoidoscopy, blood cultures, and stool cultures to rule out other pathophysiological causes. The Rome IV and Manning Criteria are also used.

Define the Rome IV Diagnostic Criteria for Functional Gastrointestinal Disorders and the Manning Criteria.

Rome IV:

_____
_____
_____
_____
_____

Manning Criteria: _____

_____
_____
_____
_____
_____

Medical Management:

_____
_____
_____
_____
_____
_____
_____

Medication Management:

_____
_____
_____
_____
_____
_____
_____

Section II. Application Exercise 2

The client is diagnosed with irritable bowel syndrome. The nurse knows that treatment for the disease is symptom based. Create a care plan for the client based on the following nursing diagnosis:

Nursing Diagnosis	Patient Outcomes	Interventions	Evaluation
Chronic pain related to spasms and increased motility			
Ineffective coping related to psychosocial effects of IBS			
Ineffective health maintenance related to living with chronic disease			
Alteration in nutrition related to disease process			

Section III. Inflammatory Bowel Disease

Case Scenario: A 25-year-old female is admitted to the emergency department with left lower quadrant pain. She has a history of watery bowel movements that have bright red blood every 2–3 hours for the last 36 hrs. Four years ago, she was diagnosed with inflammatory bowel disease and at that time was hospitalized. Her current medications are only prn in which she takes Metamucil. IV started and labs drawn on client.

Client is to be transferred to unit. Emergency department nurse calls to report to the unit:

Vitals: T: 100.1, P: 108, R: 20, BP: 110/70, Ht: 5′5″, Wt: 118 lbs. Skin warm, dry. Lungs clear.

IV D5W at 125ml/hr into left forearm; two bloody BMs during the last 3 hours in the emergency department; no urine passed since admission.

Labs: Hgb: 9.8 gm, HCT: 29%, Potassium: 2.8, BUN: 24.

NPO except only ice chips, up in chair qid.

Orders: Esophagogastroduodenoscopy (EGD) and colonoscopy today. NG tube to low intermittent suctioning to be inserted if vomiting persists with irrigation of NG tube prn.

Inflammatory Bowel Disease

Define:

_____

_____

_____

_____

Tidbit

Inflammatory bowel disease occurs during the teenage years and young adulthood but can have a second peak in the 6th decade.

Classifications

Ulcerative Colitis:

_____
_____
_____
_____

Crohn's:

_____
_____
_____
_____

Etiology/Pathophysiology:

_____
_____
_____
_____
_____
_____
_____
_____

Manifestations Crohn's:

_____
_____
_____
_____
_____
_____
_____
_____
_____
_____
_____

Manifestations Ulcerative Colitis:

_____
_____
_____
_____

_____
_____
_____
_____

Pattern of Inflammation for Crohn's:

_____
_____
_____
_____
_____
_____
_____
_____
_____

Pattern of Inflammation for Ulcerative Colitis:

_____
_____
_____
_____
_____
_____
_____
_____
_____
_____

Section III. Application Exercise 1

The EGD reveals that the client has Crohn's disease. The following diagnoses applies to the client: <u>Diarrhea</u>, <u>deficient fluid volume</u>, <u>imbalanced nutrition</u>, <u>ineffective coping</u>. Using the diagram below, create a concept map for nursing management for Crohn's disease.

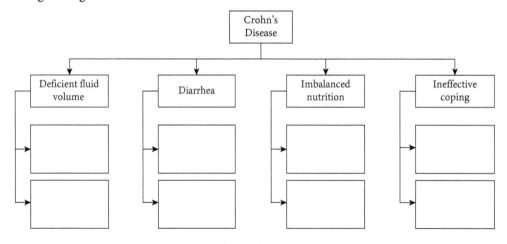

Diagnostic Studies:

_____

_____

_____

_____

_____

_____

_____

_____

Medical Management:

_____

_____

_____

_____

_____

_____

_____

_____

Medications:

_____

_____

_____

_____

_____

_____

_____

_____

Section III. Application Exercise 2

Nutrition is a big concern for the client. Create a teaching plan that focuses on the nutritional aspect of inflammatory bowel disease.

Teaching Plan

Diet	Vitamins	Foods to Avoid

Nursing Management

Assessment:

_____
_____
_____
_____
_____
_____
_____
_____
_____

Diagnosis:

_____
_____
_____
_____

Planning/Interventions:

_____
_____
_____
_____

Evaluation:

_____
_____
_____
_____

Gerontological Considerations:

_____
_____
_____
_____

Section IV. Celiac Disease

Case Scenario: Ms. Tripp, a 22-year-old, is seen in the health care provider's office. She has complaints of diarrhea and vomiting for a week, abdominal pain, weight loss of 15 lbs in one month, fatigue, dehydration, and severe thirst. She has a family history of diabetes type 1, celiac disease, rheumatoid arthritis, and psoriasis. She has a personal history of celiac disease, chronic constipation, weight loss, and abdominal pain associated with her celiac disease diagnosis. She states, "I have had this disease for quite some time now, but I have a hard time managing it. I don't talk about it too much."

   Nursing assessment reveals:

   Vitals: T: 99.6, P: 90, R: 22, BP: 136/78, O_2 saturation: 98%. Lungs clear, skin dry.

Celiac Disease

Define:

_____
_____
_____

Foods High in Gluten:

_____
_____
_____
_____
_____

> *Tidbit*
>
> Gluten, which is related to the cause of celiac disease, is not only found in foods, but also in some hair and skin products.

Etiology/Pathophysiology:

_____
_____
_____
_____

Manifestations:

_____
_____
_____
_____

Diagnostic Tests:

_____
_____
_____
_____

Section IV. Application Exercise

Based on the client's manifestations, select a priority diagnosis and decide in what order you would implement your care.

Priority Problem   #1   #2   #3   #4

Nursing Interventions:

   a. Develop a trusting relationship.
   b. Refer client to dietitian.
   c. Refer to support group for celiac disease.
   d. Encourage client to choose gluten-free choices when dining out.

Nursing Management:

_____
_____
_____
_____
_____
_____

Section V. Diverticulosis/Diverticulitis

Case Scenario: A 56-year-old male is seen in the emergency department with complaints of left lower quadrant pain. The client states he has not had an appetite for the last several days and feels bloated. He also states he has had some loose stools that look like there are small amounts of mucus and blood. The client has a history of smoking and NSAID use.

Vitals: T: 101, P: 92, R: 24, BP: 146/86, O_2 saturation: 98%.

Diverticulitis/Diverticulosis

Define:

Diverticula: _____

Diverticulosis: _____

Diverticulitis: _____

Etiology/Pathophysiology:

_____
_____
_____
_____

Manifestations:

_____
_____
_____
_____

Diagnostic Studies:

_____
_____
_____
_____

Management:

_____
_____
_____
_____

> *Tidbit*
>
> Diverticula are not the same as polyps. Diverticula are small pouches that are open to the lumen of the bowel. Polyps are benign tumors derived from cells lining the large intestine.

Surgical Management:

_____

_____

_____

_____

Section V. Application Exercise

Lab results reveal leukocytosis, elevated C-reactive protein. CT scan and colonoscopy show inflamed, infected pouches. The client is diagnosed with diverticulitis. Implement your plan of care for this client.

Nursing Diagnosis:

1. Acute pain related to _____

2. Knowledge deficit related to _____

Assessments:

Vital Signs:

_____

Labs:

_____

I&O:

_____

Pain:

_____

_____

_____

Antibiotics:

_____

_____

_____

Dietary Recommendations:

_____

_____

_____

Evaluation:

_____

_____

_____

Section VI. Intestinal Obstruction

Case Scenario: Mr. Wilson, a 55-year-old male, is admitted to the unit with a diagnosis of small bowel obstruction. The health care provider has ordered an NG tube to low continuous suction that is draining dark brown drainage. There is some abdominal distention, and upon auscultation, the nurse finds hyperactive bowel sounds in the right lower and upper quadrants and hypoactive bowel sounds in the left lower and upper quadrants. The client has an IV infusing of D5/0.45NS with 20 of KCl at 75ml/hr. Currently, the client is complaining of nausea and has just vomited 75 ml of brownish emesis.

Vitals: T: 98.9, P: 92, R: 26, BP:146/78. Pulse oximetry: 97%.

Intestinal Obstruction

Define:

_____

_____

_____

_____

Tidbit

Digested food particles must travel through 25 ft or more of intestines as part of normal digestion. Intestinal obstruction can put a stop to this.

Mechanical:

_____

_____

Types:

_____

_____

Nonmechanical:

_____

_____

Types:

_____

_____

Manifestations:

_____

_____

_____

_____

Diagnostic Studies:

_____

_____

_____

_____

Management:

_____

_____

_____

_____

Section VI. Application Exercise

You are assigned to care for the client on the unit. From the above assessment, as you begin to plan your care, prioritize what you would do to care for the client.

_____ Introduce yourself to the client.

_____ Provide oral hygiene care.

_____ Assess and measure abdominal girth.

_____ Make sure client is in semi-Fowler's position.

_____ Assess NG tube placement and suction is intact.

_____ Take vital signs.

Section VII. Anorectal Disorders

Case Scenario: Mr. Rogers, a 38-year-old bank manager, is seen in the health care provider's office with his wife with complaints of rectal bleeding. He has a history of about 4 weeks of streaks of bright red blood in his stools and scant blood on the toilet paper when he wipes. He has had some pain and itching around the anal area after bowel movements. His wife states she told him it was probably hemorrhoids and told him to use some witch hazel on his rectal area to relieve the pain and irritation. The condition seemed to have improved, but he noticed an unusually large smear of bright red blood on the toilet paper this morning, the day of his visit. The bleeding was not associated with pain. Further questioning revealed that he states he has sluggish bowel movements and has moved his bowels no more than 3 times a week. He voiced that he does strain at times and stools are solid but not hard. There was no change in bowel habits and denies any family history of colonic cancer. He has always enjoyed good health.

Vital signs: T: 98.6, P: 90, BP: 136/72. Oxygen saturation: 100%.

Anorectal Disorders

Hemorrhoids:

Define: _____
_____
_____
_____

Etiology/Pathophysiology:

Internal: _____
_____
_____

External: _____
_____
_____

> *Tidbit*
>
> Anorectal disorders are a common reason for visits to both primary care physicians and gastroenterologists. These disorders are varied and include benign conditions such as hemorrhoids to more serious conditions such as malignancy.

Section VII. Application Exercise 1

Determine the cause of Mr. Rogers's bleeding and diagnostic studies that may be ordered.

Causes: _____
_____

Diagnostic Studies: _____
_____
_____

Manifestations:

_____

_____

_____

_____

Nursing Management:

_____

_____

_____

_____

Section VII. Application Exercise 2

Mr. Rogers has been diagnosed with internal and external hemorrhoids. Develop a teaching plan for the client to manage his condition.

Teaching Instructions
Medications
Signs and symptoms to notify health care provider
Sitz baths
Diet
Bowel movements

Anal Fissure

Define: _____

_____

_____

_____

Etiology/Pathophysiology:

_____
_____
_____
_____

Manifestations:

_____
_____
_____
_____

Nursing Management:

_____
_____
_____
_____

Anal Fistula

Define: _____
_____
_____
_____

Etiology/Pathophysiology:

_____
_____
_____
_____

Manifestations:

_____
_____
_____
_____

Nursing Management:

_____
_____
_____
_____

Critical Thinking Questions

1. A patient being admitted with an acute exacerbation of ulcerative colitis complains of crampy abdominal pain and passing 10 or more bloody stools a day. The nurse initially will plan to

   a. administer IV metoclopramide (Reglan)

   b. place the patient on NPO

   c. administer cobalamin (vitamin B12) injections

   d. teach the patient about total colectomy surgery

2. A patient has a new diagnosis of Crohn's disease after having frequent diarrhea and a weight loss of 15 lbs over 2 months. The nurse will plan to teach about

   a. medication use

   b. fluid restriction

   c. enteral nutrition

   d. activity restrictions

3. A patient with diverticulosis has a large bowel obstruction. The nurse will monitor for

   a. referred back pain

   b. metabolic alkalosis

   c. projectile vomiting

   d. abdominal distention

4. Which question from the nurse would help determine if a patient's abdominal pain might indicate irritable bowel syndrome (IBS)?

   a. Have you been passing a lot of gas?

   b. What foods affect your bowel patterns?

   c. Do you have any abdominal distention?

   d. How long have you had abdominal pain?

5. Which breakfast choice indicates a patient's good understanding of information about a diet for celiac disease?

   a. Oatmeal with nonfat milk

   b. Whole wheat toast with butter

   c. Bagel with low-fat cream cheese

   d. Corn tortilla with scrambled eggs

Chapter 8

Hepatic, Biliary, and Pancreatic Alterations

Introduction

This chapter will examine hepatic, biliary, and pancreatic alterations and the disease processes related to them.

T HE LIVER SERVES as the body's cleansing organ, with many functions. It stores and filters blood. It produces bile and is responsible for clotting factors of II, VII, IX, and X, and prothrombin. It also plays a role in removing clotting factors to prevent clotting. In addition, the liver assists in the metabolism of carbohydrates, fats, and proteins. As a storage function, it stores vitamins A, D, E, and K and iron. When the liver is not able to perform these functions, disease develops.

The purpose of the biliary system is to transport bile, which is a necessary digestive enzyme that breaks down fats, from the liver to the gallbladder, where it is stored and then on to the duodenum. If there is inflammation, blockage to the ducts or infection to the gallbladder, several disorders can occur.

Learning Objectives of This Chapter

Upon completion of this chapter, the student should be able to:

- Discuss the pathophysiology and clinical manifestations of hepatic, biliary, and pancreatic problems.
- Describe age-related changes in the hepatic, biliary, and pancreatic systems.
- Describe common hepatic, biliary, and pancreatic problems.
- Describe the nursing process in which hepatic, biliary, and pancreatic problems may occur.
- Identify common hepatic, biliary, and pancreatic medications.
- Identify important components of a subjective and objective hepatic, biliary, and pancreatic health history.

Section I. Hepatic

Case Scenario: A 23-year-old female visits her health care provider's office after 2 days with an elevated temperature and flu-like symptoms. She states she has taken ibuprofen every 4 hours but has not had relief. The client states this morning she noticed that her eyes "seem yellow." She states that her bowel movements are normal, but her stools seem "lighter" and her urine is dark. There is no significant health history, and the client states she has been feeling fine since this current illness. Her family history is positive for cardiovascular disease from her father. She expressed to the health care provider that she had the Hepatitis B injection as a little girl, so she thought that she would not need another hepatitis injection. She states she has traveled to South Africa recently with a group from her college. She states she enjoyed her trip and participated in swimming in the local river and other activities during the trip.

Vitals: T: 99.9, P: 78, R: 20, BP: 118/76.

Self Study Guide

COMPLETE THE FOLLOWING as you listen to the lecture and/or refer to your textbook.

Tidbit

The incidence and prevalence of hepatitis is worldwide. The goal of Healthy People 2020 is to reduce hepatitis infections through education.

Hepatitis

Define:

_____
_____
_____

Etiology/Pathophysiology:

_____
_____
_____
_____

Types of Hepatitis:

_____
_____
_____
_____
_____
_____
_____
_____

Manifestations:

_____
_____
_____
_____

Diagnostic Tests:

_____

_____

_____

_____

_____

_____

_____

_____

_____

_____

Section I. Application Exercise 1

Looking at the above assessment of the client, what type of hepatitis does this patient have?

_____

Why?

_____

_____

_____

_____

Medical Management:

_____

_____

_____

_____

_____

_____

_____

_____

Diet and Activity:

_____

_____

_____

_____

_____

_____

_____

_____

_____

Surgical Management:

_____
_____
_____
_____
_____
_____
_____
_____
_____

Section I. Application Exercise 2

The client has been diagnosed with hepatitis A. She is confused as to how she could have gotten hepatitis since she had an injection for hepatitis B as a little girl. Develop a nursing diagnosis for this situation and a teaching plan for the patient.

NURSING DIAGNOSIS

_____

Teaching Plan

Activity	Nutrition	Importance of Vaccinations to Prevent Hepatitis A and B

Nursing Management

Assessment:

_____
_____
_____
_____
_____
_____
_____

Diagnosis:

_____
_____
_____
_____

Planning:

_____
_____
_____
_____
_____
_____
_____
_____

Interventions:

_____
_____
_____
_____
_____
_____
_____
_____
_____

Evaluation:

_____
_____
_____
_____
_____
_____
_____
_____

Section II. Liver Cirrhosis

Case Scenario: A 50-year-old male is admitted to the emergency department accompanied by his wife. The client presents with complaints of feeling fatigued and abdominal distention. His wife states he has been forgetting things lately and acting strangely. She says she noticed weight gain in the client, but his appetite is poor. The patient has a history of drinking for over 20+ years. He states he stopped about 2 years ago but states he has not been feeling well for a long time. Nursing assessment reveals:

Vitals: T: 99.0, P: 90, R: 24, BP: 146/88. Pulse oximetry: 97%.

Physical assessment: skin jaundiced, sclera of eyes is yellow, red palms bilaterally, lesions to left lower leg, abdominal girth 50cm.

Past Medical History: hypertension, history of alcohol abuse, pneumonia 5 years ago. Total knee replacement 25 years ago.

Liver Cirrhosis

Define:

_____
_____
_____
_____
_____

Etiology/Pathophysiology:

_____
_____
_____
_____
_____
_____
_____
_____
_____

Manifestations:

Early:

_____
_____
_____
_____

Late:

_____
_____
_____
_____

Jaundice:

_____
_____
_____

Skin Lesions:

_____

_____

_____

Hematologic Problems:

_____

_____

_____

Endocrine Problems:

_____

_____

_____

Peripheral Neuropathy:

_____

_____

_____

Section II. Application Exercise 1

The client is admitted to the unit and the health care provider orders the following laboratory test: liver function studies, prothrombin time, serum albumin levels, liver ultrasound. The client and his wife are questioning what these tests are for. Explain the purpose of the lab test and what the values indicate related to liver cirrhosis.

Liver Function Test	Purpose	Normal/Abnormal Values
AST		
ALT		
Alkaline phosphatase		
GGT		
Prothrombin Time		
Serum Albumin		
Liver Ultrasound		

Complications

Portal Hypertension:

_____
_____
_____

Esophageal Varices:

_____
_____
_____

Management of Esophageal Varices:

_____
_____
_____
_____

Balloon Tamponade

Define:

_____
_____

Sengstaken-Blakemore Tube:

_____
_____

Minnesota Tube:

_____
_____

Linton-Nachlas Tube:

_____
_____

Management of Bleeding:

_____
_____

_____

Peripheral Edema:

_____

_____

_____

Ascites:

_____

_____

_____

Management of Ascites:

_____

_____

_____

_____

Hepatic Encephalopathy:

_____

_____

_____

Hepatorenal Syndrome:

_____

_____

_____

Diagnostic Studies:

_____

_____

_____

_____

_____

_____

_____

Medical Management:

_____
_____
_____
_____
_____
_____
_____
_____
_____
_____

Drug Therapy:

_____
_____
_____
_____

Nutritional Therapy:

_____
_____
_____
_____

Shunting Procedures:

_____
_____

Portacaval Shunt:

_____
_____
_____
_____

Distal Splenorenal Shunt:

_____
_____
_____
_____

Section II. Application Exercise 2

The lab results reveal that the client has liver cirrhosis. The health provider orders the following: sodium restriction of 250 mg/day, Aldactone 100 mg daily, Furosemide 10 mg daily, Lactulose 30 ml bid, 3000 cal/day protein-restricted diet.

The following nursing diagnoses apply to the client:

- Imbalanced nutrition: less than body requirements
- Excess fluid volume
- Impaired skin integrity
- Deficient knowledge

Develop a care plan that addresses the above diagnoses in a priority order. Incorporate the health care provider's orders in your plan of care.

Prioritized Nursing Diagnosis	Client Outcome	Interventions with Rationale	Evaluation

Section III. Liver Trauma

Case Scenario: A 35-year-old patient presents to the emergency department with a stab wound to his right upper quadrant from a fight in a bar. The patient has lost a large amount of blood and places his T-shirt over the stab wound site trying to control the bleeding.

Vitals: P: 102, R: 28, BP: 90/56. The client has guarding pain to the area of the stab wound and abdomen is firm and tense. Skin is pale and cool. Labs reveal elevated liver enzymes.

Liver Trauma

Define:

_____

_____

_____

_____

Etiology/Pathophysiology:

_____

_____

_____

_____

_____

_____

_____

_____

Diagnostic Studies:

_____

_____

_____

_____

_____

_____

_____

_____

> *Tidbit*
>
> Because of the vasculature, size, and location of the liver, it is the most vulnerable organ to trauma in the abdominal cavity.

Section III. Application Exercise

The following orders have been written for the client:

- Administer blood, 3 units of packed red cells _____
- Administer antibiotics _____
- Monitor vital signs _____
- Obtain labs: CBC, serum electrolytes, liver function tests _____
- Start IV of 0.9% NS at 125 ml/hr _____
- Obtain CT scan _____
- Measure abdominal girth _____
- I&O _____

Prioritize in what order you would implement the above orders.

Medical Management:

_____
_____
_____
_____
_____
_____
_____
_____

Nursing Management

Assessment:

_____
_____
_____
_____
_____
_____

Diagnosis:

_____
_____
_____
_____
_____
_____

Planning/Interventions:

_____
_____
_____
_____
_____
_____
_____

Evaluation:

_____
_____

_____
_____
_____
_____
_____
_____
_____

Section IV. Cholelithiasis/Cholecystitis

Case Scenario: Connie, a 42-year-old female, is seen in the emergency department with complaints of abdominal pain that has lasted for the last 2 days. She states the pain comes and goes and sometimes radiates to her back.

Vitals: T: 100.1, P: 92, R: 24, BP: 138/86.

Physical assessment reveals pain on palpation to right upper quadrant as the patient takes deep breaths; skin yellow.

Liver function test, CBC, and ultrasound and endoscopic retrograde cholangiopancreatography (ERCP) are ordered.

Cholelithiasis

Define:

_____
_____
_____

Cholecystitis

Define:

_____
_____
_____
_____
_____
_____
_____

Tidbit
Women who are multiparous, over 40, or postmenopausal on hormone replacement therapy are at higher risk for cholelithiasis.

Section IV. Application Exercise

ERCP and ultrasound reveal cholecystitis. Develop a concept map for this medical diagnosis.

Nursing diagnosis	Risk factors	Complications	Nursing interventions

Cholecystitis

Pathophysiology	Signs & Symptoms	Diagnostic procedures

Medical Management:

_____
_____
_____
_____

Lithotripsy:

_____
_____
_____
_____

Cholecystectomy:

_____
_____
_____
_____

Post-op Nursing Management

Teaching:

_____
_____
_____
_____

T-Tube Management:

_____
_____
_____
_____

Diet:

_____
_____
_____
_____

Symptoms to report to health care provider:

_____
_____
_____
_____

Evaluation:

_____
_____
_____
_____

Section V. Pancreatitis

Case Scenario: A 45-year-old client presents to the immediate care center with complaints of left upper quadrant pain that has gotten worse over the last few days. He states the pain gets worse when he eats. The client states he has had some nausea and vomiting with this pain.

Vitals: T: 99.9, P: 98, R: 26, BP: 118/70.

Other assessment findings:

- Dyspnea, crackles in lungs, cyanosis
- Tender abdomen with hypoactive bowel sounds

- Bluish discoloration around the flank
- Periumbilical bruising
- Yellow skin

Pancreatitis

Define:

_____
_____
_____
_____

Etiology/Pathophysiology:

_____
_____
_____
_____

Manifestations:

Acute:

_____
_____
_____
_____
_____
_____
_____
_____
_____

Chronic:

_____
_____
_____
_____
_____
_____
_____
_____

> *Tidbit*
>
> The most common cause of pancreatitis is gallbladder disease and alcohol abuse.

Complications:

_____
_____
_____
_____
_____
_____
_____
_____
_____

Section V. Application Exercise 1

The client has orders for a laboratory test to rule out acute pancreatitis. For each laboratory value, state whether the test would be elevated or decreased and the rationale for the result.

Serum Laboratory Test	Level	Rationale
Albumin		
Amylase		
AST		
ALT		
Calcium		
Direct Bilirubin		
Lipase		
WBC		

Diagnostic Studies

Other Tests:

_____
_____
_____
_____

Medical Management:

_____
_____
_____
_____
_____
_____
_____
_____

Section V. Application Exercise 2

Acute pancreatitis has been identified as the diagnosis. Several medications are used to manage acute pancreatitis. For each medication, list the rationale for its use.

Medication	Rationale for Use
Opioid narcotics—morphine sulfate	
Anticholinergic agents	
Spasmolytics	
H2 antagonist or proton pump inhibitors	
Pancreatic enzymes	
Antibiotics	
Octreotide	

Nutritional Management:

_____

_____

_____

_____

Section V. Application Exercise 3

The following nursing diagnoses apply to the client:

Acute pain, ineffective breathing pattern, knowledge deficit, imbalanced nutrition.

Put each diagnosis in priority order and develop a plan of treatment that addresses each.

Nursing Diagnosis	Patient Outcomes	Interventions	Evaluation

Surgical Management for Chronic Pancreatitis:

_____
_____
_____
_____
_____
_____
_____
_____
_____
_____

Evaluation:

_____
_____
_____
_____

Critical Thinking Questions

1. Which assessment information will be most important for the nurse to report to the health care provider about a patient with acute cholecystitis?

   a. The patient's urine is bright yellow.

   b. The patient's stools are tan colored.

   c. The patient has increased pain after eating.

   d. The patient complains of chronic heartburn.

2. The nurse is caring for a 73-year-old man who has cirrhosis. Which data obtained by the nurse during the assessment will be of most concern?

   a. The patient's hands flap back and forth when the arms are extended.

   b. The patient complains of right upper-quadrant pain with palpation.

   c. The patient has ascites and a 2-kg weight gain from the previous day.

   d. The patient's skin has multiple spider-shaped blood vessels on the abdomen.

3. Which information given by a 70-year-old patient during a health history indicates to the nurse that the patient should be screened for hepatitis C?

   a. The patient had a blood transfusion in 2005.

   b. The patient used IV drugs about 20 years ago.

   c. The patient frequently eats in fast-food restaurants.

   d. The patient traveled to a country with poor sanitation.

4. The nurse is planning care for a 48-year-old woman with acute severe pancreatitis. The highest priority patient outcome is

    a. maintaining normal respiratory function.

    b. expressing satisfaction with pain control.

    c. developing no ongoing pancreatic disease.

    d. having adequate fluid and electrolyte balance.

Chapter 9

Renal/Urological Alterations

Introduction

This chapter will examine renal and urological alterations and the disease processes related to them.

T HE KIDNEYS' PRIMARY function is to remove waste from the body, maintain fluid and electrolyte balance, and play a role in regulating acid-base balance. If the kidneys are not functioning properly, illness occurs and death can occur. It is important to implement measures to correct any kidney malfunction promptly in order to maintain renal function.

Learning Objectives of This Chapter

Upon completion of this chapter, the student should be able to:

- Discuss the pathophysiology and clinical manifestations of renal and urological problems.
- Identify important components of a subjective and objective renal and urological health history utilizing critical thinking and therapeutic communication to support rapid focused assessment leading to accurate collaborative care.
- Describe common urinary elimination health problems.
- Describe the nursing process in which urinary elimination problems may occur.
- Identify common renal and urinary medications.

Section I. Polycystic Kidney Disease

Case Scenario: A 48-year-old man is in the outpatient center with complaints of right lower back and abdominal pain. The client also is complaining of headache. The client has a history of type 2 diabetes and hypertension.

Vitals: T: 100.1, P: 90, R: 26, BP: 152/92.

Physical exam reveals bilateral enlarged kidneys and costovertebral angle tenderness. A CT scan, IV pyelogram, and MRI findings are suggestive of polycystic kidney disease.

Self Study Guide

Complete the following as you listen to the lecture and/or refer to your textbook.

Polycystic Kidney Disease

Define:

_____

_____

_____

_____

Etiology/Pathophysiology:

_____

_____

_____

_____

_____

_____

_____

_____

Manifestations:

_____

_____

_____

_____

_____

Section I. Application Exercise 1

Match the lab test with the results associated with PKD.

Hemoglobin/Hematocrit	Elevated due to impaired renal elimination
Plasma Creatinine/BUN	Anemia due to decreased production of erythropoietin
Plasma Potassium	Elevated causing fluid retention
Urinalysis/Urine Culture	Elevated due to impairment of renal clearance
Plasma Calcium	Decreased due to renal damage causing impairment of conversion of vitamin D to its active form
Plasma Sodium	Elevated due to impaired renal clearance of waste products
Plasma Phosphorus	Potential for UTI due to compression of cyst that impairs elimination

Medical Management:

_____

_____

_____

_____

_____

_____

_____

Section I. Application Exercise 2

Lab and diagnostic results confirm polycystic kidney disease.
The following orders are given to the nurse for the client:

Report any manifestations of infection   _____

Instruct on dietary and fluid restrictions   _____

Administer antihypertensives as ordered   _____

Administer antibiotics as ordered   _____

Administer pain meds as ordered   _____

Obtain vital signs   _____

Administer O_2 at 2l via nasal cannula   _____

Prioritize the orders that must be carried out

Nursing Management

Assessment:

_____

_____

_____

_____

Diagnosis:

_____

_____

_____

_____

Planning:

_____

_____

_____
_____
_____
_____
_____

Interventions:

_____
_____
_____
_____
_____
_____
_____

Evaluation:

_____
_____
_____
_____

Section II. Pyelonephritis

Case Scenario: A 26-year-old female is seen in the health care provider's office with complaints of painful urination, back pain, incontinence. She verbalized feeling nauseated. The client states she has noticed a pinkish tinge in her urine and feels feverish. The client has a history of UTIs and usually just drinks cranberry juice and lets it pass.

  Vital signs reveal: T: 100.6, P: 88, R: 26, BP: 98/60.

  Assessment: Enlarged kidneys noted on palpation and guarding exhibited by client.

  Labs ordered: Urinalysis, urine culture, CBC, CT scan.

Pyelonephritis

Define:

_____
_____
_____
_____

Etiology/Pathophysiology:

_____
_____

Tidbit

Young women are most often affected by pyelonephritis, mostly likely due to sexual activity and increased susceptibility of UTIs, the major risk factor associated with the disease.

_____
_____

Manifestations:

_____
_____
_____
_____

Diagnostic Tests:

_____
_____
_____
_____

Medical Management:

_____
_____
_____
_____
_____
_____

Section II. Application Exercise

Lab results confirm pyelonephritis. The following nursing diagnosis applies to the client:
Infection, ineffective therapeutic regimen management, impaired urinary elimination, deficient knowledge.
Create your plan of care in priority order using the above nursing diagnosis.

Nursing Diagnosis	Patient Outcome	Interventions	Evaluation

Nursing Management

Assessment:

_____
_____
_____
_____

Diagnosis:

_____

_____

_____

_____

Planning:

_____

_____

_____

_____

Interventions:

_____

_____

_____

_____

_____

_____

Evaluation:

_____

_____

_____

_____

Section III. Acute and Chronic Glomerulonephritis

Case Scenario: Mr. Smith, a 35-year-old male, is seen in the emergency department with a complaint of abdominal and lower back pain for a couple of weeks. The client states he had strep throat before the pain started. Client has generalized edema and states he has not been able to urinate effectively, but when he does, his urine appears dark.

Vital signs: T: 99.9, R: 22, P: 90, BP: 168/96.

Labs ordered: Urinalysis, urine culture, CBC, renal function studies.

Acute Glomerulonephritis

Define:

_____

_____

_____

Tidbit

Glomerulonephritis is the third leading cause of renal failure in the United States.

Etiology/Pathophysiology:

_____

_____

_____

_____

Manifestations:

_____

_____

_____

_____

Section III. Application Exercise 1

The assessment and labs reveal acute glomerulonephritis.
Describe the significance of the client's recent strep throat infection on the diagnosis of acute glomerulonephritis.

_____

_____

_____

_____

Medical Management:

_____

_____

_____

_____

_____

_____

_____

_____

Section III. Application Exercise 2

An early course of treatment is initiated for the client. Since the treatment is based on cause, the client will be treated with penicillin for the post-streptococcal glomerulonephritis. The client's other diagnosis will also need to be treated. Please indicate the rationale for the other treatments prescribed for the client.

Treatment	Rationale
Diuretics	
Antihypertensives	
Corticosteroids	
Restriction of dietary protein	

Nursing Management

Assessment:

_____

_____

_____

_____

_____

_____

_____

Diagnosis:

_____

_____

_____

_____

Planning:

_____

_____

_____

_____

_____

_____

_____

Interventions:

_____

_____

_____

_____

_____

_____

_____

Evaluation:

_____

_____

_____

_____

_____

_____

_____

Section III. Application Exercise 3

Differentiate between acute and chronic glomerulonephritis.

	Acute Glomerulonephritis	Chronic Glomerulonephritis
Causes		
Symptoms		
Diagnostic Tests		
Treatment		

Section IV. Renal Trauma

Case Scenario: A 40-year-old male was brought into the emergency department after being involved in a motor vehicle accident. The client is responsive and states he has pain in his abdominal and back areas. Assessment reveals a palpable mass and hematuria. CT scan, ultrasound and renal arteriogram are done, revealing a pelvic fracture which perforated the right kidney.

> *Tidbit*
>
> Renal trauma usually occurs due to the lack of bone to protect the area as compared to other organs.

Renal Trauma

Define:

_____
_____
_____
_____

Etiology/Pathophysiology:

_____
_____
_____
_____

Medical Management:

_____
_____
_____
_____
_____
_____
_____
_____

Section IV. Application Exercise 1

Renal trauma is graded according to the extent of the injury. Complete the table below with the manifestations of each grade.

GRADE	MANIFESTATION
1	
2	

3	
4	
5	

Section IV. Application Exercise 2

Based on the client's symptoms, the following diagnoses apply:

Acute pain, impaired urinary elimination.

Complete a care plan for the two diagnoses, including all nursing management aspects below.

Nursing Management

Assessment:

_____
_____
_____
_____
_____
_____
_____

Client Outcomes:

_____
_____
_____
_____
_____
_____
_____

Interventions:

_____
_____
_____
_____
_____
_____
_____

Evaluation:

_____
_____
_____
_____
_____
_____
_____

Section V. Acute and Chronic Kidney Injury

Case Scenario: Mrs. Lewis, a 50-year-old female, is seen in her primary health care provider's office. She has had several days of little urine output. Her daughter, who is accompanying her, states she has been short of breath when walking around the house and seems to be forgetting things. The client has 3+ edema in bilateral lower extremities.

Vital signs: T: 98.9, P: 100, R: 26, BP: 96/65.

Labs obtained reveal increased potassium, phosphorus, BUN/creatinine, decreased calcium, sodium, and pH.

Results reveal acute kidney injury.

Acute Kidney Injury (AKI)

Tidbit
Acute kidney injury is reversible but has a high mortality rate.

Define:

_____
_____
_____
_____

Etiology/Pathophysiology:

_____
_____
_____
_____

Three Major Categories:

Prerenal:

_____
_____
_____

Intrarenal:

_____

_____

_____

Postrenal:

_____

_____

_____

Section V. Application Exercise 1

Looking at the manifestation exhibited by the client, which phase of AKI is the client in?

_____

Phases of Acute Kidney Injury:

Initiating Phase:

_____

_____

_____

Oliguric Phase:

_____

_____

_____

Diuretic Phase:

_____

_____

_____

Recovery Phase:

_____

_____

_____

Section V. Application Exercise 2

Kidney disease has many manifestations. In the chart below, list the causes of each manifestation.

Manifestation	Cause
Urine volume decreases	
Fluid overload	
Increased potassium	
Anemia	
Metabolic acidosis	
Decreased sodium	
Increased BUN	
Decreased calcium/ increased phosphorus	
Increased creatinine	

Medical Management:

_____
_____
_____
_____
_____
_____
_____

Medications:

_____
_____
_____
_____

Nutrition:

_____

_____

_____

_____

RIFLE Classification for Staging Acute Kidney Injury

GFR criteria   *Urine Output Criteria*

<u>R</u>isk   _____

<u>I</u>njury   _____

<u>F</u>ailure   _____

<u>L</u>oss   _____

<u>E</u>nd-stage renal disease   _____

Section V. Application Exercise 3

Hyperkalemia is a severe complication of AKI. Explain why elevated potassium levels are harmful to the client's condition.

Hyperkalemia Effects:

_____

_____

_____

_____

_____

Section V. Application Exercise 4

Create a concept map for your plan of care for the client with acute kidney injury.

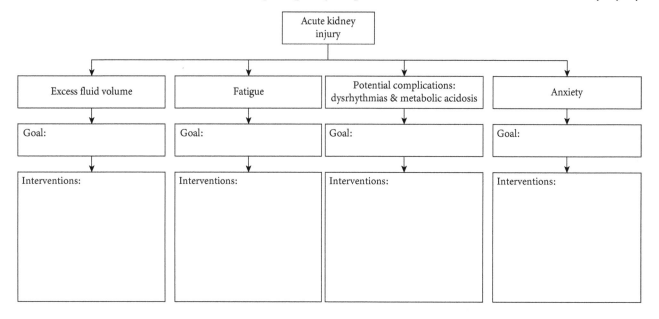

Case Scenario: A 65-year-old client with type 2 diabetes, hypertension, and coronary artery disease is seen by the diabetic educator for teaching on the management of her diabetes. She states she has been short of breath and her legs feel heavy due to increased swelling in her lower legs. She also complains of itching in her extremities.

Vital signs: T: 98.9, R: 26, P: 98, BP: 168/94, oxygen saturation: 96%.

Height: 5′3″, Weight: 198 lbs.

Labs drawn at the office visit: H&H, serum creatinine, GFR, Hgb A1C, serum electrolytes, lipid profile, arterial blood gas, urine for protein.

> **Tidbit**
>
> Chronic kidney disease is responsible for premature death and is responsible for a high economic price from both the private and public sectors.

Chronic Kidney Disease (CKD)

Define:

_____

_____

_____

_____

Section V. Application Exercise 5

What risk factors for chronic kidney disease does the client have?

_____

_____

_____

_____

Manifestations:

_____

_____

_____

_____

Section V. Application Exercise 6

The client's results are as follows:

Test	Client's Results	Target Range
Hemoglobin	9.0 g/dL	11.7–15.5 g/dL
Hematocrit	30%	36–48%
Creatinine	2.6 mg/dL	0.5–1.2 mg/dL
GFR	58 mL/min/1.73 m^2	90–120 mL/min/1.73 m^2
BUN	24 mg/dl	8–21 mg/dl
HbgA1c	8.0%	<7.0%
LDL	148 mg/dL	<100 mg/dL
HDL	42 mg/dL	>40 mg/dL (preferably >60 mg/dL)
Arterial pH	7.30	7.35–7.45
Serum CO_2	20	23–29 mEq/L
Calcium	8.0 mg/dL	8.2–10.2 mg/dL
Phosphorus	4.4 mg/dL	2.5–4.5 mg/dL
Potassium	5.2 mEq/L	3.5–5.0 mEq/L
Serum Sodium	134 mEq/L	135–145 mEq/L
Urine Protein	9.6 g/dl	6–8 g/dL

Looking at the client's lab results, chronic renal failure is confirmed. Using the information below, indicate a treatment plan that should be implemented for each condition.

Treatment (Control of):

Hyperkalemia:

_____

_____

_____

_____

_____

Hypertension:

_____

_____

_____

Renal Osteodystrophy:

_____
_____
_____
_____
_____

Hypocalcemia:

_____
_____
_____
_____
_____

Hyperparathyroidism:

_____
_____
_____
_____

Anemia:

_____
_____
_____
_____

Dyslipidemia:

_____
_____
_____

Medications:

_____
_____
_____

Nutrition:

_____

_____

_____

_____

_____

Surgical Management

Renal Transplant:

_____

_____

_____

_____

_____

_____

_____

_____

Complications:

_____

_____

_____

_____

_____

_____

_____

_____

Section V. Application Exercise 7

The following diagnoses apply to the client:

Excess fluid volume, disturbed thought processes, fatigue, risk for dysrhythmias.

Using the above diagnosis, create a plan of care for the client.

Nursing Management

Assessment:

_____

_____

_____

_____

_____

_____

_____

Client Outcomes:

_____
_____
_____
_____
_____
_____
_____

Interventions:

_____
_____
_____
_____
_____
_____
_____

Evaluation:

_____
_____
_____
_____
_____
_____
_____

Section VI. Renal Replacement Therapies

Case Scenario: A 60-year-old female is admitted to the hospital with a history of end-stage renal disease, hypertension, and diabetes. She presents with fatigue, confusion, and lethargy. She has bilateral 2+ edema to bilateral lower extremities. Lungs have course crackles bilaterally.

Vitals: T: 98.8, P: 90, R: 28, BP: 168/90, pulse oximetry: 96%.

Labs: H&H, BUN, serum creatinine, creatinine clearance, serum electrolytes, urine for C&S, urinalysis, and HgbA1c.

Renal Replacement Therapies

Tidbit

The process of renal replacement therapy depends on the processes of diffusion and filtration.

Define:

_____
_____
_____

_____

_____

_____

Section VI. Application Exercise 1

The client's condition continues to deteriorate. Her creatinine clearance is 8, and she has become increasingly uremic as evidenced by confusion, BP 170/92, and an increase in edema in hands and feet. She continues to have crackles bilaterally in her lungs. The health care provider is preparing the client for hemodialysis.

Use the table below to compare the advantages and disadvantages of peritoneal dialysis and hemodialysis.

Advantages	Disadvantages
Peritoneal	
Hemodialysis	

Hemodialysis

Define:

_____

_____

_____

Vascular Access:

_____
_____
_____
_____
_____
_____
_____

Hemodialysis Process:

_____
_____
_____
_____
_____
_____
_____

Continuous Renal Replacement Therapy

Define:

_____
_____
_____
_____
_____
_____
_____
_____
_____

Peritoneal Dialysis

Define:

_____
_____
_____
_____
_____
_____
_____
_____

Contraindications:

_____
_____
_____
_____
_____
_____
_____

Complications:

_____
_____
_____
_____
_____
_____
_____

Section VI. Application Exercise 2

The client had an arteriovenous fistula placed 3 days and is to receive hemodialysis via a percutaneous cannula to her right subclavian vein until the fistula is healed and is ready for use. She will have outpatient dialysis 3 days a week. The client verbalizes that she is not sure if she will be able to get to her appointments and states, "I am not sure how to take care of myself and I am worried about being able to afford dialysis."

Develop a teaching plan using the nursing diagnosis to address the issues the client is verbalizing.

Nursing Diagnosis	Teaching Plan
Deficient knowledge related to disease process	

Impaired nutrition related to dietary management of end-stage renal disease	
Anxiety r/t management of disease process	
Ineffective coping related to financial management of disease	
Risk for infection related to arteriovenous fistula and percutaneous cannula	

Section VII. Urinary Tract Infections, Urolithiasis, Urinary Incontinence

Case Scenario: A 20-year-old female is seen in the outpatient clinic with complaints of painful urination for the last 2 days. She states she has also been feeling nauseated and has not been able to keep food down.

Vital signs: T: 100.1, P: 90, R: 24, BP: 96/60.

Labs: Urinalysis, urine culture.

Urinary Tract Infections (UTIs)

Define:

_____

_____

_____

_____

_____

> **Tidbit**
>
> The annual cost of treating UTIs is over $1 billion and is the most common reason for outpatient visits.

Section VII. Application Exercise 1

The client's labs reveal leukocytosis, *Escherichia coli*, and red blood cells in the urine. Urine appears cloudy. The client is diagnosed with an uncomplicated UTI. The client asked how this could have occurred. Describe the risk factors and possible causes of urinary tract infections.

Etiology/Pathophysiology

Complicated UTIs:

_____

_____

_____

Uncomplicated UTIs:

_____

_____

_____

Manifestations:

_____

_____

_____

_____

Medical Management:

_____

_____

_____

_____

Section VII. Application Exercise 2

The following diagnoses apply to the client:
Altered urinary elimination, knowledge deficit, acute pain.
Prioritize and develop a plan of care for the client.

Nursing Management

Assessment:

_____

_____

_____

_____

_____

_____

_____

_____

Planning:

_____

_____

_____

_____

_____

_____

_____

_____

Interventions:

_____

_____

_____

_____

_____

_____

_____

_____

Evaluation:

_____

_____

_____

_____

_____

_____

_____

Case Scenario: A 55-year-old male presented to the emergency department with complaints of back, groin, and flank pain. The client rates his pain as a 10 out of 10. He states the pain is constant and has had an episode of vomiting before he came to the emergency department. He denies shortness of breath or chest pain.

Vital signs: T: 98.9, P: 88, R: 24, BP: 136/78. Pulse oximetry: 99%.

Diagnostic test: CT scan and urinalysis ordered. Urine shows some hematuria.

Urolithiasis

Etiology/Pathophysiology:

_____

_____

_____

_____

_____

_____

_____

> *Tidbit*
>
> Urinary stones affect 12 per 10,000 people in the United States and occur more in males.

Section VII. Application Exercise 3

The client's urinalysis shows a UTI with the presence of *Pseudomonas* bacteria, CT scan shows a struvite stone measuring about 5mm to right ureter. List the causes and treatment for each type of stone.

Types	Causes	Treatment
Calcium Oxalate		
Calcium Phosphate		
Struvite		
Uric Acid		
Cystine		

Medical Management

Acute Attack:

_____
_____
_____
_____

Endourologic Procedures

Cystoscopy: _____
_____
_____

Cystolitholathopaxy: _____
_____
_____

Cystoscopic

Lithotripsy: _____
_____
_____

Surgical Therapy

Percutaneous

Nephrolithotomy: _____
_____
_____
_____
_____
_____

Section VII. Application Exercise 4

Since the stone is only 5mm in size, the health care provider does not recommend any invasive treatment. Create a teaching plan to assist the client in passing the stone.

Interventions	Teaching Plan
Medications Analgesics Antiemetics Alpha Blockers	
Fluids	
Straining Urine	
Kidney Stone Prevention	

Etiology/Pathophysiology:

_____
_____
_____
_____

Medical Management:

_____
_____
_____
_____
_____
_____
_____

Nursing Management

Assessment:

_____
_____
_____
_____
_____
_____
_____

Diagnosis:

_____
_____
_____
_____

Planning:

_____
_____
_____
_____
_____
_____
_____

Interventions:

_____
_____
_____
_____
_____
_____
_____

Evaluation:

_____
_____
_____
_____
_____
_____

Incontinence

Define:

_____

_____

_____

_____

Section VII. Application Exercise 5

For each type of incontinence, list the cause or risk factors and manifestations.

Incontinence Type	Cause or Risk Factor	Manifestations
Stress		
Urge		
Mixed		
Overflow		
Functional		
Reflex		

Etiology/Pathophysiology:

_____

_____

_____

_____

Medical Management

Stress:

_____

_____

_____

_____

Urge:

_____

_____

_____

_____

Reflex:

_____

_____

_____

_____

Overflow:

_____

_____

_____

_____

Functional:

_____

_____

_____

_____

Surgical Management

Stress:

_____

_____

_____

_____

Urge:

_____

_____

_____

_____

Reflex:

_____
_____
_____
_____

Overflow:

_____
_____
_____
_____

Functional:

_____
_____
_____
_____

Nursing Management

Assessment:

_____
_____
_____
_____
_____
_____

Diagnosis:

_____
_____
_____
_____

Planning:

_____
_____
_____
_____

Interventions:

_____
_____
_____
_____
_____
_____
_____
_____

Evaluation:

_____
_____
_____
_____
_____
_____
_____
_____

Section VIII. Benign Prostatic Hypertrophy

Case Scenario: A 76-year-old male is seen in the health care provider's office with complaints of difficulty urinating. He states he feels like he needs to urinate but that it has been difficult to begin urine flow, even with straining. He also states that even when he starts a urine stream, it stops and starts and there is dribbling. History reveals his job as a retired accountant, smoking x 30 years, diet high in fats, and a sedentary lifestyle.

   Vital signs: T: 99.6, P: 88, R: 26, BP: 146/86, pulse oximetry: 98%.

   Diagnostic Test: Prostate-specific antigen (PSA), digtial rectal exam (DRE).

Benign Prostatic Hypertrophy (BPH)

Tidbit
Enlargement of the prostate and prostate cancer are independent of each other.

Define:

_____
_____
_____
_____

Etiology/Pathophysiology:

_____
_____

_____
_____

Risk Factors:

_____
_____
_____
_____

Manifestations

Irritative Symptoms:

_____
_____
_____
_____

Obstructive Symptoms:

_____
_____
_____
_____

Complications:

_____
_____
_____
_____

Diagnostic Studies

Digital Rectal Exam:

_____
_____
_____
_____

Prostate-Specific Antigen (PSA):

_____
_____

Transrectal Ultrasound:

_____

_____

Uroflowmetry:

_____

_____

Cystoscopy:

_____

_____

Section VIII. Application Exercise 1

The DRE and PSA indicate the patient has benign prostatic hypertrophy.

The client is started on 5 alpha reductase inhibitors and an alpha blocker. Develop a teaching plan for the client on these medications.

5 Alpha Reductase Inhibitors	Mechanism of Action
1. _____ 2. _____ 3. _____ 4. _____ 5. _____	
Alpha Blockers _____ _____ _____	**Mechanism of Action**

Alternative Management:

_____

_____

_____

_____

Medical Management:

_____
_____
_____
_____

Minimally Invasive

Transurethral Microwave Therapy (TUMT):

_____
_____

Transurethral Needle Ablation (TUNA):

_____
_____

Laser Prostatectomy:

_____
_____

Intraprostatic Urethral Stents:

_____
_____

Invasive Therapies

Transurethral Resection (TURP):

_____
_____

Transurethral Incision of the Prostate (TUIP):

_____
_____

Nursing Management

Assessment:

_____
_____

_____

_____

_____

_____

_____

Diagnosis:

_____

_____

_____

_____

Planning/Interventions:

_____

_____

_____

_____

Section VIII. Application Exercise 2

After several weeks on the prescribed medication regimen, the client continues to have urinary frequency and urgency problems. The health care provider schedules a transurethral resection of the prostate (TURP). List the preop care the nurse will give to the client.

Preop TURP Care

_____

_____

_____

_____

The client has had a TURP and vitals are: T: 98.6, P: 86, R: 22, BP: 146/86, pulse oximeter: 100%. The client is sent to the unit with a 3-way urinary catheter to gravity with continuous irrigation with normal saline for clots. He states he is having some pain in his lower abdomen. Prioritize the flowing orders to care for the client along with the rationale for your interventions.

Get client up in chair after dinner   _____

Take vital signs   _____

Assess pain level   _____

Give pain medication for bladder spasms   _____

Empty catheter drainage bag   _____

Assess irrigation system   _____

Evaluation   _____

_____

_____

_____

_____

_____

Critical Thinking Questions

1. It is most important that the nurse ask a patient admitted with acute glomerulonephritis about

   a. history of kidney stones

   b. recent sore throat and fever

   c. history of high blood pressure

   d. frequency of bladder infections

2. A 28-year-old male patient is diagnosed with polycystic kidney disease. Which information is most appropriate for the nurse to include in teaching at this time?

   a. Complications of renal transplantation

   b. Methods for treating severe chronic pain

   c. Discussion of options for genetic counseling

   d. Differences between hemodialysis and peritoneal dialysis

3. Which assessment finding for a patient who has just been admitted with acute pyelonephritis is most important for the nurse to report to the health care provider?

   a. Complaint of flank pain

   b. Blood pressure 90/48 mm Hg

   c. Cloudy and foul-smelling urine

   d. Temperature 100.1°F (57.8°C)

4. When a patient with acute kidney injury (AKI) has an arterial blood pH of 7.30, the nurse will expect an assessment finding of

   a. persistent skin tenting.

   b. rapid, deep respirations.

   c. bounding peripheral pulses.

   d. hot, flushed face and neck.

Chapter 10

Endocrine Alterations

Introduction

This chapter will examine endocrine alterations and the disease processes related to them.

T HE ENDOCRINE SYSTEM consists of a network of glands that make hormones that work along with the nervous system. This coordination assists with sustaining bodily functions, including growth and development, sexual function, metabolism, and blood sugar regulation. Any alteration in these functions causes a dysfunction of the glands and the hormones they secrete. If the problem is of a primary nature, there is an actual dysfunction of the gland itself. If there is a secondary problem, the anterior pituitary is malfunctioning. A tertiary problem is due to a hypothalamus problem. If the target tissue doesn't respond to hormones, this is a quaternary problem.

Learning Objectives of This Chapter

Upon completion of this chapter, the student should be able to:

- Discuss the pathophysiology and clinical manifestations of imbalance of endocrine problems.
- Describe common endocrine health problems.
- Describe the nursing process in which endocrine problems may occur.
- Identify common endocrine medications.

Section I. Overview of the Endocrine System

Self Study Guide

Complete the following as you listen to the lecture and/or refer to your textbook.

Endocrine System

Define:

_____
_____
_____
_____

The Hypothalamus

Location:

_____
_____

Secretes:

_____
_____
_____
_____

The Pituitary Gland

Location:

_____
_____

Anterior pituitary secretes the following hormones:

_____
_____
_____
_____

Posterior pituitary stores and releases:

_____
_____
_____
_____

The Thyroid Gland

Location:

_____
_____

Secretes the following hormones:

_____
_____
_____
_____

The Parathyroid Glands

Location:

_____
_____

Secrete the following hormones:

_____
_____
_____
_____

The Adrenal Glands

Location:

_____
_____

Adrenal Cortex

Secretes the following hormones:

_____
_____
_____
_____

Adrenal Medulla

Location:

_____

_____

Secretes the following hormones:

_____

_____

_____

_____

The Pancreas

Location:

_____

_____

The islets have three types of cells:

The ALPHA cells secrete _____

The BETA cells secrete _____

The DELTA cells secrete _____

Exocrine Function:

_____

_____

_____

_____

The Gonads

Female

Location:

_____

_____

Male

Location:

_____

_____

Secrete the following hormones:

_____

_____

Section I. Application Exercise 1

Use the concept word list to fill in the concept map.

Endocrine Concept **Word List**

Ovary	Calcium from bones
Testes	Thymosins
Kidney	Insulin
Hypothalamus	Immune Function
Stomach	Glucagon
Heart	T3/T4
Adrenal	Contractions (labor)
Thyroid	Calcium from bones
Thymus	Uptake of glucose
Parathyroid	Female development
Pituitary	Raises blood sugar
Pineal body	Male development
Pancreas	Maintains blood pressure
Melatonin	Testosterone
PTH	Sex hormones
ADH	Stabilizes blood glucose
Oxytocin	Male, female function
FSH	Energy
LH	Epinephrine
ACTH	Aldosterone
GH	Increases heart rate
PRL	Sperm and egg production
Milk production	Growth
Stress hormone	Vasopressin water balance
Sleep cycles	Calcitonin
Estrogen cortisol	Maintains blood glucose
	Regulates sex hormones

Endocrine Concept Map

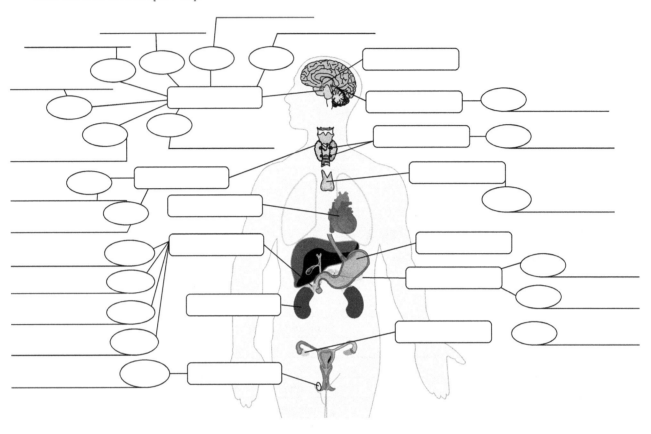

Common Laboratory Procedures

Hormone Levels Assay:

_____
_____
_____
_____

Hormone Levels of T3/T4:

_____
_____
_____
_____

Radioactive Iodine Uptake (RAI):

_____
_____
_____
_____

Thyroid Scan:

_____

_____

_____

_____

Fasting Blood Glucose:

_____

_____

_____

_____

Glucose Tolerance Test:

_____

_____

_____

_____

Glycosylated Hemoglobin A1C

_____

_____

_____

_____

_____

_____

_____

_____

Section I. Application Exercise 2

Match the laboratory test with its significance of being increased or decreased with the hyper/hypo function disorder.

Test	Significance
Sodium (135–145mEq/L)	(increased/decreased) in diabetes insipidus (increased/decreased) in SIADH (increased/decreased) in hypercortisolism (increased/decreased) in hypocortisolism (increased/decreased) in hyperaldosteronism (increased/decreased) in hypoaldosteronism

Potassium (3.5–5.0mEq/L)	(increased/decreased) in hypercortisolism (Addison's) (increased/decreased) in hypercortisolism (Cushing's)
Calcium (8.2–10.2 mg/dL)	(increased/decreased) in hypoparathyroidism (increased/decreased) in hyperparathyroidism (increased/decreased) by thyrocalcitonin from the thyroid gland
Magnesium (1.6–2.6 mg/dL)	(increased/decreased) in hypoparathyroidism
Phosphorus (2.5–4.5 mg/dL)	(increased/decreased) in hypoparathyroidism (increased/decreased) in hyperparathyroidism
Ionized Calcium (4.6–5.3 mg/dL)	(increased/decreased) in hypoparathyroidism (increased/decreased) in hyperparathyroidism
Glucose (65–99 mg/dL)	(increased/decreased) in diabetes mellitus (increased/decreased) in hypercortisolism
Cortisol (5–25 mcg/dL—mornings) (3–16 mcg/dL—afternoons)	(increased/decreased) in hypercortisolism (Addison's) (increased/decreased) in hypercortisolism (Cushing's)
Free T3 (triiodothyronine) (2.6–4.8 pg/ml)	(increased/decreased) in hypothyroidism (increased/decreased) in hyperthyroidism
Total T3 (triiodothyronine) (70–204 ng/dL)	(increased/decreased) in hypothyroidism (increased/decreased) in hyperthyroidism
Free T4 (thyroxine) (0.8–1.5 ng/dL)	(increased/decreased) in hypothyroidism (increased/decreased) in hyperthyroidism
Total T4 (thyroxine) (4.6–12 mcg/dL)	(increased/decreased) in hypothyroidism (increased/decreased) in hyperthyroidism
Thyroid stimulating hormone (TSH) (0.5–8.9 MIU/mL)	(increased/decreased) in hypothyroidism (increased/decreased) in hyperthyroidism (increased/decreased) in secondary or tertiary hypothyroidism (increased/decreased) in secondary or tertiary hyperthyroidism
Urine specific gravity (1.005–1.030)	(increased/decreased) in DI (increased/decreased) in SIADH
Vitamin D (20–100 ng/dL)	(increased/decreased) hypoparathyroidism (increased decreased) hyperparathyroidism

Section II. Disorders of the Endocrine Glands—Pituitary

Define:

1. HYPER- _____

2. HYPO- _____

Case Scenario: A 40-year-old male presents at the outpatient clinic accompanied by his wife. The client states he has noticed that his voice has changed and he has experienced an increase in his shoe size. The wife states he stopped wearing his wedding ring because he told her it doesn't fit anymore. The client also complains of feeling tingling and numbness in his hands. He denies any pain but states, "I have occasional headaches and I just do not feel like myself; it is uncomfortable. This has been going on for several months now." Assessment reveals broad forehead and enlarged nose, lips, and ears; eyes bulging.

Vital signs: T: 99, P: 84, R: 24, BP: 166/100. Ht: 5'7", Wt: 178 lbs.

Labs ordered: Hormonal studies—ACTH stimulation test, TSH, growth hormone, CT scan, and MRI of the head.

Anterior Pituitary

Hypopituitarism

Define:

_____
_____
_____
_____

Causes: _____

Pathophysiology:

_____
_____
_____
_____

Tidbit

Hypopituitarism is a rare disorder and usually affects the anterior pituitary.

Section II. Application Exercise 1

Because of a decrease in growth hormone, glucocorticoid, mineralocorticoid, and decreased secretion of ACTH, the client will be at risk for several problems. Formulate at least <u>three</u> nursing diagnoses and develop a plan of care for each related to pituitary hypofunction.

Nursing Diagnosis	Client Goals	Interventions	Rationale

Section II. Application Exercise 2

For each hormone, list the manifestation seen for hypopituitarism.

Hormone	Manifestations
Thyroid-stimulating Hormone (TSH)	
Decreased T3 & T4	
Adrenocorticotropic Hormone (ACTH)	
Decreased glucocorticoids	
Decreased mineralocorticoids	
Growth Hormone	
Follicle-stimulating Hormone	
Males	
Females	
Luteinizing Hormone	
Males	
Females	

Hyperpituitarism

_____
_____
_____
_____

Causes: _____

Pathophysiology: _____

Assessment Findings:

_____
_____
_____
_____

Section II. Application Exercise 3

The client's CT scan and MRI are positive for pituitary tumor. Labs reveal hypersecretion of growth hormone. Thyroid studies are within normal limits. The client has been diagnosed with acromegaly and is scheduled for a transsphenoidal hypophysectomy. Develop a teaching plan that will assist the patient in understanding the procedure and your nursing responsibility during this procedure.

Hypophysectomy

Procedure:

_____
_____
_____
_____
_____

Nursing Interventions

Preop Care:

_____
_____
_____
_____
_____
_____

Nursing Interventions

Postop Care:

_____
_____
_____
_____
_____
_____
_____
_____

Posterior Pituitary

Diabetes Insipidus

Define:

Central:

_____
_____
_____
_____

Nephrogenic:

_____
_____
_____
_____

Pathophysiology:

_____
_____
_____
_____
_____
_____

Assessment Findings:

_____
_____
_____
_____

Tidbit

The posterior pituitary is not glandular as is the anterior pituitary. It is made up of mostly nerve cells from the hypothalamus.

Diagnostic Tests:

_____

_____

_____

_____

Nursing Interventions:

_____

_____

_____

_____

Syndrome of Inappropriate Antidiuretic Hormone (SIADH)

_____

_____

Causes: _____

Pathophysiology: _____

Assessment Findings:

_____

_____

Section II. Application Exercise 4

Diabetes insipidus (DI) causes an excessive water loss that results in hemoconcentration. Syndrome of Inappropriate Antidiuretic Hormone (SIADH) causes water overload. Indicate what happens to the lab tests below as a result of these posterior pituitary disorders.

Significance	
Hematocrit	SIADH
Normal Value:	DI
Serum Sodium	SIADH
Normal Value:	DI
Urine-specific Gravity	SIADH
Normal Value:	DI

Diagnostic Tests:

_____

_____

_____

_____

Nursing Interventions:

_____
_____
_____
_____
_____
_____
_____
_____
_____

Section III. Disorders of the Endocrine Glands—Adrenal Gland

Case Scenario: Mrs. Evans, a 30-year-old female, presents to the health care provider's office with complaints of fatigue and weight loss for several weeks. The client states she has been increasingly weak and is very irritable. She says it has been difficult to concentrate at work as a bank executive.

Vital signs: T: 98.8, P: 88 and irregular, R: 20, BP: 92/72, pulse oximetry: 97%. Ht: 5′6″, Wt: 118 lbs.

Assessment reveals: dry skin and mucus membranes, dark pigmentation on the face.

Labs ordered: Serum electrolytes, cortisol levels, CT scan, and MRI.

Addison's Disease

Adrenal Hypofunction (Insufficiency)

Define:

_____
_____
_____

Causes: _____

Pathophysiology:

_____
_____
_____
_____
_____
_____

Tidbit

The adrenal gland gets its name from its position: *ad* (near or at) + *renes* (kidneys).

Section III. Application Exercise 1

The health care provider has ordered several diagnostic studies to rule out adrenal insufficiency. Below, fill in the blanks for each test to indicate their levels with adrenal insufficiency.

Serum electrolytes	
Sodium	_____ (Increased, Decreased)
Potassium	_____ (Increased, Decreased
Glucose	_____ (Increased, Decreased)
Cortisol	_____ (Increased, Decreased)
The best time to draw a cortisol level is _____ because _____ _____	

Assessment Findings:

_____

_____

_____

_____

Section III. Application Exercise 2

Lab results indicate acute adrenal insufficiency. The health care provider has ordered the following:

- IV fluids of 100 mg of hydrocortisone in 100 mL of 0.9% NS solution at 10 ml/hr.
- Monitor vital signs q 4 hrs.
- Labs for serum electrolytes to be drawn this evening.

Prioritize how you would carry out the following nursing actions:

_____ Place bed in lowest position

_____ Administer hydrocortisone

_____ Ensure vascular access for IV administration

_____ Assess vital signs

_____ Draw lab specimen

Section III. Application Exercise 3

The client's condition is stabilized, and she is being discharged home. The nurse is responsible for implementing a teaching plan for the client. Develop a discharge teaching plan for the client.

Medication management
Stress management
Lifestyle changes

Nursing Interventions:

_____
_____
_____
_____

Addisonian Crisis

_____
_____
_____
_____

Causes: _____

Treatment:

_____
_____
_____

Adrenal Cortex Hyperfunction

Cushing's Disease

_____
_____
_____
_____

Causes: _____

Pathophysiology: _____

Diagnostic Tests:

_____
_____

Assessment Findings:

_____
_____
_____
_____

Nursing Interventions:

_____
_____
_____
_____

Conn's Syndrome

_____
_____
_____
_____

Causes: _____

Pathophysiology: _____

Diagnostic Tests:

_____
_____

Assessment Findings:

_____
_____
_____
_____

Nursing Interventions:

_____
_____
_____
_____

Section III. Application Exercise 4

Cushing's and Conn's diseases cause hypersecretion of adrenal cortex hormones.

Using the diagram, create a concept map for nursing management for adrenal cortex hyperfunction disease.

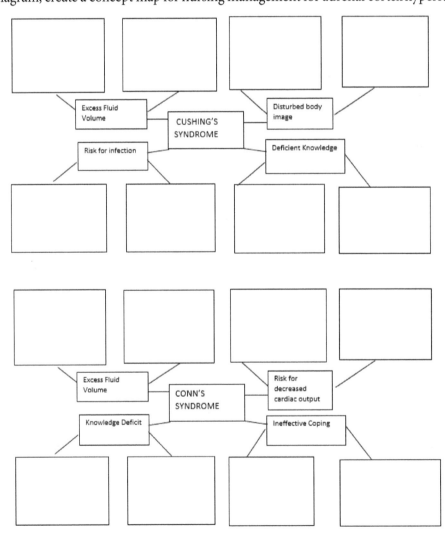

Pheochromocytoma

_____

_____

_____

_____

Causes: _____

Pathophysiology: _____

Assessment Findings:

_____

_____

_____

_____

Nursing Interventions:

_____

_____

_____

_____

Section IV. Disorders of the Endocrine Glands—Thyroid Gland

Case Scenario: A 32-year-old female presents to the health care provider's office. She states that over the last few months, she has begun to feel lethargic and very moody and at times cannot remember things. She states her bowels have become sluggish and she is constipated. Denies pain. She has a history of cardiovascular disease. Physical exam reveals puffiness around her face, dry, scaly skin, and dry thinning hair.

Vital signs: T: 97.6, P: 60, R: 16, BP: 90/70, pulse oximetry: 97%.

Labs ordered: Thyroid studies.

Hypothyroidism

_____

_____

_____

_____

Causes: _____

Pathophysiology: _____

> *Tidbit*
>
> The thyroid gland is only about 2 inches across and usually cannot be seen or felt.

Section IV. Application Exercise 1

The client's lab reveals elevated TSH (4.6), free T3 decreased (2.0), total T3 decreased (65), free T4 decreased (0.6), total T4 decreased (4.0). For each of these hormones, indicate their actions.

Hormone	Action
Thyroid-Stimulating Hormone (TSH)	
Triiodothyronine (Free T3)	
Triiodothyronine (Total T3)	
Thyroxine (Free T4)	
Thyroxine (Total T4)	

Medical Management
Hormone Replacement Therapy

Section IV. Application Exercise 2

The client is diagnosed with hypothyroidism. The health care provider gives an order for hormone replacement therapy.

Fill in the blanks.

1. The primary treatment for hypothyroid is _____ . It is the most common medication used for treatment of hypothyroidism. It is best to give the medication to the client _____ . Teaching will include telling the client that the medication must be taken for _____ and should be taken_____.

2. Why is the client's history of cardiovascular disease a concern with this medication?

_____
_____
_____
_____

Assessment Findings:

_____
_____
_____
_____

Nursing Diagnosis:

_____
_____
_____

Nursing Interventions:

_____

_____

_____

_____

Complications

Myxedema Coma

Define:

_____

_____

_____

_____

Causes: _____

Pathophysiology: _____

Assessment Findings:

_____

_____

_____

_____

Nursing Diagnosis:

_____

_____

_____

Nursing Interventions:

_____

_____

_____

_____

Hyperthyroidism

_____

_____

_____

_____

Causes: _____

Pathophysiology: _____

Medical Management

Medications

Propylthiouracil (PTU)

Mechanism of Action: _____

    Nursing Implications

_____

Methimazole (Tapazole)

Mechanism of Action: _____

    Nursing Implications

_____

Lithium Carbonate

Mechanism of Action: _____

    Nursing Implications

_____

Iodine (SSKI-saturated Solutions of Potassium Iodine)

Mechanism of Action: _____

    Nursing Implications

_____

Section IV. Application Exercise 3

An overactive thyroid puts clients in a hypermetabolic state. The following nursing diagnoses apply to hyperthyroidism:

- Decreased cardiac output
- Altered nutrition: less than body requirements
- Hyperthermia

Create a **care plan that addresses each of the nursing diagnoses.**

Nursing Diagnosis	Client Goals	Interventions	Rationale
Decreased cardiac output related to:			
Altered nutrition: less than body requirements related to:			
Hyperthermia related to:			

Complications

Thyroid Storm

Define:

_____
_____
_____
_____

Causes: _____

Pathophysiology: _____

Assessment Findings:

_____
_____
_____
_____

Nursing Diagnosis:

_____
_____
_____

Nursing Interventions:

_____
_____
_____
_____

Surgical Management

Thyroidectomy:

_____
_____
_____

Preop Care Thyroidectomy:

_____
_____

Postop Care Thyroidectomy:

_____

_____

_____

_____

_____

Section V. Disorders of the Endocrine Glands—Parathyroid Gland

Case Scenario: Mr. Davis, a 37-year-old male who had a thyroidectomy 2 days ago, is now experiencing numbness and tingling around hands, feet, and mouth. The client also complains of muscle cramps.

Vitals signs: T: 98.7, P: 88 and irregular, R: 20, BP: 90/60, pulse oximetry: 98%.

Orders given: Place patient on cardiac monitor; draw following labs: PTH, serum calcium, magnesium, and phosphorus level, and Vitamin D, tracheostomy tray at bedside.

Hypoparathyroidism

_____

_____

_____

_____

Causes: _____

Pathophysiology: _____

Chvostek's Sign: _____

Trousseau's Sign: _____

Medical Management

> ### Tidbit
> While their names are similar and they are near each other, the functions of the thyroid and parathyroid are independent of each other.

Section V. Application Exercise

The lab results reveal hypocalcemia secondary to hypoparathyroidism. Prioritize the following nursing orders for the care of the client:

Teach patient about medication regimen	_____
Check vital signs	_____
Assess cardiac monitor	_____
Administer calcium supplements	_____
Administer vitamin D	_____
Teach high-calcium/low-phosphorus diet	_____

Assessment Findings:

_____
_____
_____
_____

Nursing Diagnosis:

_____
_____
_____
_____

Nursing Interventions:

_____
_____
_____
_____

Hyperparathyroidism

_____
_____
_____
_____

Causes: _____

Pathophysiology: _____

Medical Management

Assessment Findings:

_____
_____
_____
_____

Nursing Diagnosis:

_____
_____
_____

Nursing Interventions:

_____

_____

_____

_____

Critical Thinking Questions

1. A patient is scheduled for transsphenoidal hypophysectomy to treat a pituitary adenoma. During preoperative teaching, the nurse instructs the patient about the need to

   a. cough and deep breathe every 2 hours postoperatively.

   b. remain on bed rest for the first 48 hours after the surgery.

   c. avoid brushing teeth for at least 10 days after the surgery.

   d. be positioned flat with sandbags at the head postoperatively.

2. A 40-year-old patient with suspected acromegaly is seen at the clinic. To assist in making the diagnosis, which question should the nurse ask?

   a. Have you had a recent head injury?

   b. Do you have to wear larger shoes now?

   c. Is there a family history of acromegaly?

   d. Are you experiencing tremors or anxiety?

3. A 56-year-old patient who is disoriented and reports a headache and muscle cramps is hospitalized with possible syndrome of inappropriate antidiuretic hormone (SIADH). The nurse would expect the initial laboratory results to include a(n)

   a. elevated hematocrit.

   b. increased serum chloride.

   c. decreased serum sodium.

   d. low urine specific gravity.

4. An expected patient problem for a patient admitted to the hospital with symptoms of diabetes insipidus is

   a. excess fluid volume related to intake greater than output.

   b. impaired gas exchange related to fluid retention in lungs.

   c. sleep pattern disturbance related to frequent waking to void.

   d. risk for impaired skin integrity related to generalized edema.

5. A patient who had radical neck surgery to remove a malignant tumor developed hypoparathyroidism. The nurse should plan to teach the patient about

   a. bisphosphonates to reduce bone demineralization.

   b. calcium supplements to normalize serum calcium levels.

   c. increasing fluid intake to decrease risk for nephrolithiasis.

   d. including whole grains in the diet to prevent constipation.

Figure Credit

Chapter 11

Diabetes Mellitus

Introduction

This chapter will examine diabetic alterations and the disease processes related to them.

E VEN THOUGH THE disease process of diabetes is a result of pancreatic malfunction, which is part of the endocrine system, it is a multifaceted, dynamic, and complex disease process that affects all ages, body types, and ethnic groups. It requires a level of control of blood glucose levels to maintain homeostasis.

Learning Objectives of This Chapter

Upon completion of this chapter, the student should be able to:

- Discuss the pathophysiology and clinical manifestations of the imbalance of diabetic problems.
- Identify important components of a subjective and objective diabetes health history utilizing critical thinking and therapeutic communication to support rapid focused assessment leading to accurate collaborative care.
- Describe age-related changes in the diabetic system.
- Describe diabetic health problems.
- Describe the nursing process in which diabetic problems may occur.
- Identify common diabetic medications.

Section I. Overview of Diabetes
Two Hormones Responsible for Maintaining Homeostasis

Insulin (beta cells)

_____

_____

_____

_____

Glucagon (alpha cells)

_____
_____
_____
_____

Section I. Application Exercise 1

Fill in the blanks to describe the normal process of blood glucose control.

- Normal fasting blood glucose levels should fall between _____ and _____.
- The body obtains glucose from one of three sources. They are:

1. _____ by mouth and converted to glucose through digestion and absorbed in the GI tract.

2. _____ released from glycogen stored in the muscles and liver.

3. _____ via gluconeogenesis in the liver or kidneys.

Endogenous Insulin

Define:

_____
_____
_____
_____

Section I. Application Exercise 2

Using the word list, complete the concept map on the process of blood glucose level control.

Word List

Beta cells release	Blood glucose levels decrease; insulin release decreases
Insulin	Liver takes up glucose and stores it as glycogen
Alpha cells release	Cells take up more glucose
Glucagon	Liver breaks down glycogen and releases glucose to the blood
Blood glucose levels rise; glucagon levels decrease	

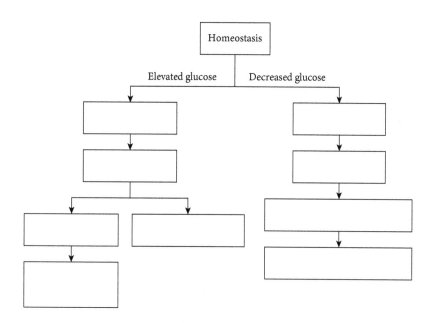

Counterregulatory Hormones

Define: What are they?

_____
_____
_____
_____

Metabolic Syndrome

List the five indications:

1. _____
2. _____
3. _____
4. _____
5. _____

Define:

_____
_____
_____
_____
_____
_____
_____

_____
_____
_____
_____

Prediabetes

Define:

_____
_____
_____
_____

Section II. Diabetes Mellitus—Type 1 and Type 2

Case Scenario: A 32-year-old male is seen in the outpatient clinic with complaints of a headache and dizziness for the last several days along with excessive thirst and urination. The client states he has a history of hypertension and takes medication daily. He states he works as an office manager for a retail company. He says his job is stressful and he doesn't do a lot of exercise outside of walking to and from the train to work. The client lives alone, eats a lot of take-out foods, and smokes a pack of cigarettes a day. Family history is positive for diabetes, renal, and heart disease.

Vital signs: T: 98.8, P: 96, R: 24, BP: 178/106, pulse oximetry: 98%.

Labs drawn: Triglycerides: 250 mg/dL; HDL 35 mg/dL, LDL 220 mg/dL, Glucose: 320 mg/dL, HgbA1C: 7.0%.

Type 2 Diabetes Mellitus

Define:

_____
_____
_____
_____

> *Tidbit*
>
> According to the CDC, more than 34 million people in the United States have diabetes, and 1 in 5 of them doesn't know they have it.

Section II. Application Exercise 1

From the information above, list the risk factors that put the client at risk for diabetes.

Risk Factors:

_____
_____
_____
_____

Etiology/Pathophysiology:

_____
_____
_____
_____
_____
_____
_____
_____
_____
_____
_____
_____

Section II. Application Exercise 2

Discuss how the four major metabolic abnormalities have a role in the development of type 2 diabetes.

1. Insulin resistance:

_____
_____
_____
_____

2. Decreased ability of the pancreas to produce insulin:

_____
_____
_____
_____

3. Inappropriate glucose production by the liver:

_____
_____
_____
_____

4. Alteration in production of hormones and cytokines by adipose tissue:

_____
_____
_____
_____

Medical Management

Diagnosis of diabetes mellitus is made through one of four methods:

1.

   _____
   _____
   _____
   _____

2.

   _____
   _____
   _____
   _____

3.

   _____
   _____
   _____
   _____

4.

   _____
   _____
   _____
   _____

Section II. Application Exercise 3

The client is diagnosed with type 2 diabetes. The health care provider has ordered a glucose monitor and education on type 2 diabetes for the client. For each topic of teaching, write the implementation and rationale for each.

Teaching Topics	Rationale
Diet	
Use of glucometer	
Exercise	
Monitoring for complications	

Goals of Diabetes Management:

_____
_____
_____
_____
_____
_____
_____
_____
_____
_____

Oral Agents (OAs) and Noninsulin Injectable Agents

Purpose:

_____
_____
_____
_____

How Do They Work?

_____

_____

_____

_____

Section II. Application Exercise 4

For each oral glucose control agent, state its mechanism of action and side effects.

Oral Agent	Mechanism of Action	Side Effects
Biguanides • Metformin		
Sulfonylureas • DiaBeta, Glynase, or Micronase (glyburide or glibenclamide) • Amaryl (glimepiride) • Diabinese (chlorpropamide) • Glucotrol (glipizide) • Tolinase (tolazamide) • Tolbutamide		
Meglitinides • Repaglinide (Prandin) • Nateglinide (Starlix)		
Thiazolidinediones • Rosiglitazone (Avandia) • Pioglitazone (Actos)		
• Alpha-glucosidase inhibitors • Miglitol (Glyset) • Acarbose (Precose)		
DDP-4 inhibitors • Januvia (Sitagliptin) • Galvus (Vildagliptin) • Onglyza (Saxagliptin) • Tradjenta (Linagliptin)		
SGLT-2 inhibitors • Dapagliflozin (Farxiga) • Canagliflozin (Invokana) • Empagliflozin (Jardiance)		

Dietary Management:

_____

_____

_____

_____

_____
_____
_____
_____
_____
_____
_____
_____
_____
_____

Exercise Management:

_____
_____
_____
_____
_____
_____
_____
_____
_____
_____
_____
_____
_____
_____
_____
_____
_____
_____
_____

Case Scenario: A 40-year-old male client presents to the emergency department. He has had diabetes type 1 for the last 10 years. He states his blood sugar has been high constantly for the last 3 days. He states he has been busy with work and dealing with family issues and had not taken his insulin as scheduled. When the health care provider asked how he is managing his diabetes, he said that he has an old glucometer that seems to be inaccurate so he does not check his blood sugars as he should. The client states he "adjusts his insulin" based on how he feels. History reveals that the client was hospitalized initially with the diagnosis of type 1 diabetes and had a blood glucose level of 400 mg/dL. He has been on and continues to use glargine 55 units daily and Aspart per sliding scale if blood glucose levels are over 300 mg/dL 3 times a day. The client states he tries to eat three times a day, but depending on the day, he may skip a meal.

Vital signs: T: 98.8, P: 98, R: 28 and rapid, BP: 100/68, pulse oximetry: 97%.

Other assessment findings: Fruity-odor breath, increased urinary output, complaints of feeling thirsty and hungry.

Labs ordered: Hgb A1c, random blood glucose level, arterial blood gases, urine for ketones, serum electrolytes.

Type 1 Diabetes Mellitus

Define:

_____
_____
_____
_____

Etiology/Pathophysiology:

_____
_____
_____
_____
_____
_____
_____
_____
_____
_____
_____
_____

Section II. Application Exercise 5

Describe the manifestations the client is experiencing as a result of his elevated blood glucose levels.

Hypotension:

_____
_____
_____
_____

Respirations:

_____
_____
_____
_____

Excessive urination, thirst, and hunger:

_____
_____
_____

Medical Management

Diagnostic Test

Oral Glucose Tolerance Test:

_____
_____
_____

Fasting Plasma Glucose:

_____
_____
_____

Hemoglobin A1C:

_____
_____
_____

Self-Monitoring Blood Glucose:

_____
_____
_____
_____

Continuous Blood Glucose Monitoring:

_____
_____
_____
_____

Section II. Application Exercise 6

The client's lab results are: HgbA1C, 11.3%; random blood glucose level, 300 mg/dL; urine positive for ketones; ABG, pH 7.30; HCO_3, 18mEq/L; PCO_2: 20mEq/L; sodium, 132mEq/L; potassium, 3.3mEq/L; chloride, 106mEq/L; and anion gap, 10.8mEq/l. The client has been diagnosed with diabetic ketoacidosis. The client is admitted to the medical unit.

The health care provider gives the following orders:

1. Administer 0.9%NS w/20mEq of KCL @100 ml/hr.

2. Give IV insulin, regular at 0.14u/kg/hr and titrate until serum glucose reaches 250 mg/dl.

Prioritize the five nursing interventions the nurse would do to care for the client:

Perform a body system physical assessment	
Orient client to unit	
Assess IV site	
Begin IV therapy	
Obtain vital signs	

Section II. Application Exercise 7

The client's blood glucose has decreased to 200 mg/dL and the IV insulin is discontinued. The client is to be discharged with orders for insulin: 5 units of regular insulin and 10 units of NPH insulin q a.m. The health care provider also orders diabetic teaching for the client.

The following diagnoses apply to the client:

Knowledge deficit, risk for injury, anxiety, altered nutrition, ineffective health maintenance, risk for altered blood glucose levels, risk for peripheral neurovascular dysfunction.

From the above diagnoses, select a priority nursing diagnosis and list the interventions and rationale for your diagnosis.

Nursing Diagnosis	Interventions	Rationale
	1. 2. 3. 4.	

Section III. Blood Glucose Management

Exogenous (Injected) Insulin

Purpose:

_____
_____
_____
_____

Rapid-acting Synthetic Insulin Analogs

	Onset	Peak	Duration	Purpose
Humlog/Lispro				
Novolog/Aspart				
Apidra/Glulisine				

Short-acting Regular Insulin

	Onset	Peak	Duration	Purpose
Regular Humulin/Novolin				

Intermediate-acting

	Onset	Peak	Duration	Purpose
NPH				

Long-acting Insulin

	Onset	Peak	Duration	Purpose
Lantus, Toujeo, Basaglar/Glargine				
Levermir/Detemir				
Degludec/Tresiba				

Storage of Insulin:

_____
_____
_____
_____
_____
_____

Insulin Administration:

_____
_____
_____
_____
_____
_____
_____
_____
_____
_____
_____

Insulin Pump:

_____
_____
_____
_____
_____
_____

Problems Associated with Insulin Therapy

Local Inflammatory Reactions:

_____
_____
_____
_____
_____

Lipodystrophy:

_____

_____
_____
_____
_____
_____

Section IV. Complications

Hypoglycemia:

_____
_____
_____
_____

Section IV. Application Exercise

Using the word list, complete the concept maps for the dawn phenomenon and the Somogyi effect.

- Results in higher fasting blood glucose levels in a.m.
- Natural release of counterregulatory hormones
- Counterregulatory hormones are released to increase blood glucose
- Liver releases glucose stores to increase blood glucose levels
- Insulin dose given at bedtime
- Body does not have enough insulin to control glucose increase
- Blood glucose levels drop
- Blood glucose level rises

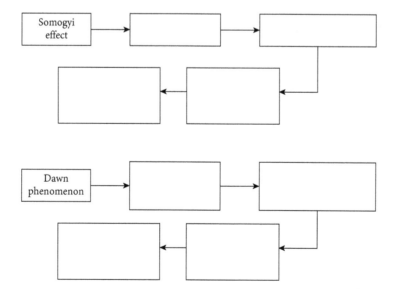

Discuss how to prevent each.

Somogyi Effect:

_____
_____
_____
_____

Dawn Phenomenon:

_____
_____
_____
_____

Panaceas Transplant:

_____
_____
_____
_____
_____
_____
_____
_____
_____
_____
_____
_____

Section V. Acute and Chronic Complications
Diabetic Ketoacidosis (DKA)

Define:

_____
_____
_____
_____

Manifestations:

_____
_____
_____
_____

Management/Nursing Care:

_____
_____
_____
_____
_____
_____
_____
_____
_____
_____
_____
_____
_____

Hyperosmolar Hyperglycemic Syndrome (HHS)

Define:

_____
_____
_____
_____

Manifestations:

_____
_____
_____
_____

Management/Nursing Care:

Define:

_____
_____
_____
_____

Manifestations:

_____
_____
_____
_____
_____

_____
_____
_____

Management/Nursing Care:

_____
_____
_____
_____

Section V. Application Exercise 1

Match the manifestation with the acute complication for diabetes.

Diabetic ketoacidosis (DKA)	Hyperosmolar hyperglycemic syndrome (HHS)
___ ___ ___ ___ ___	___ ___ ___ ___ ___

1. A medical emergency

2. Bicarbonate levels greater than 15 mEq/L

3. Blood glucose levels greater than 250 mg/dL

4. May be managed on an outpatient basis if fluid/electrolytes are not severe

5. Insulin is given immediately via IV infusion

6. Blood glucose greater than 600 mg/dL

7. Profound dehydration

8. IV administration is directed toward correcting hyperglycemia and hyperketonemia

9. Electrolytes are monitored and replaced as needed

10. Bicarbonate levels less than 18 mEq/L

Section V. Application Exercise 2

Complete the following on the "Rule of 15":

After checking _____ _____ _____ with your glucometer, if the level is under _____, consume _____ grams of _____; wait _____ minutes, then recheck _____ _____. If the blood glucose is still _____, consume another _____ grams of _____ and recheck _____ later.

_____
_____
_____

_____
_____
_____

Chronic Complications

Angiopathy:

_____
_____
_____
_____

Macrovascular Complications:

_____
_____
_____
_____
_____
_____
_____
_____

Risk Factors:

_____
_____
_____
_____

Microvascular Complications:

_____
_____
_____
_____
_____
_____
_____

Diabetic Retinopathy:

_____
_____
_____

_____
_____
_____
_____
_____
_____

Treatment:

_____
_____
_____
_____
_____
_____
_____
_____
_____

Diabetic Nephropathy:

_____
_____
_____
_____
_____
_____
_____
_____

Diabetic Peripheral Neuropathy:

_____
_____
_____
_____
_____
_____
_____
_____
_____
_____
_____

Autonomic Neuropathy

Gastrointestinal:

_____
_____
_____
_____

Sexual Dysfunction:

_____
_____
_____
_____

Urinary Problems:

_____
_____
_____
_____

Skin Problems:

_____
_____
_____
_____

Hypertension:

_____
_____
_____
_____

Gerontological Considerations

_____
_____
_____
_____
_____
_____
_____
_____
_____

Critical Thinking Questions

1. What describes the primary difference in treatment for diabetic ketoacidosis (DKA) and hyperosmolar hyperglycemic syndrome (HHS)?

    a. DKA requires administration of bicarbonate to correct acidosis.

    b. Potassium replacement is not necessary in management of HHS.

    c. HHS requires greater fluid replacement to correct the dehydration.

    d. Administration of glucose is withheld in HHS until the blood glucose reaches a normal level.

2. The patient with diabetes has a blood glucose level of 248 mg/dl. Which manifestations in the patient would the nurse understand as being related to this blood glucose level? (*Select all that apply.*)

    a. Headache

    b. Unsteady gait

    c. Abdominal cramps

    d. Emotional changes

    e. Increase in urination

    f. Weakness and fatigue

3. Following the teaching of foot care to a patient with diabetes, the nurse determines that additional instructions are needed when the patient makes which statement?

    a. "I should wash my feet daily with soap and warm water."

    b. "I should always wear shoes to protect my feet from injury."

    c. "If my feet are cold, I should wear socks instead of using a heating pad."

    d. "I'll know if I have sores or lesions on my feet because they will be painful."

4. The patient with type 2 diabetes has had trouble controlling his blood glucose with several OAs but wants to avoid the risks of insulin. The HCP told him a medication will be prescribed that will increase insulin synthesis and release from the pancreas, inhibit glucagon secretions, and slow gastric emptying. The nurse knows this is which medication that will have to be injected?

    a. Dopamine receptor agonist, bromocriptine (Cycloset)

    b. Dipeptidyl peptidase-4 (DDP-4) inhibitor, sitagliptin (Januvia)

    c. Sodium-glucose co-transporter 2 (SGLT2) inhibitor, canagliflozin (Invokana)

    d. Glucagon-like peptide-1 receptor agonist, exenatide extended release (Bydureon)

Chapter 12

Musculoskeletal Alterations

Introduction

This chapter will examine musculoskeletal alterations and the disease processes related to them.

T HE MUSCULOSKELETAL SYSTEM is the second largest system in the body and gives it the ability to move. The bones of the body make up the skeletal system. This system is the main storage for calcium and phosphorus. The cartilage, tendons, joints, ligaments, and other connective tissue that binds tissues and organs together make up the muscular system. This system keeps bones in place and plays a role in movement through contracting and pulling on bones that allow standing, walking, running, and grabbing. Joints, by way of the connective tissues of muscles, allow motion of different bones throughout the body. The cushion, which is cartilage, prevents bones from rubbing directly on each other. There are diseases and various disorders which may affect the function of the musculoskeletal system. These diseases and disorders make movement difficult and impair mobility.

Learning Objectives of This Chapter

Upon completion of this chapter, the student should be able to:

- Discuss the pathophysiology and clinical manifestations of the imbalance of musculoskeletal problems.
- Identify important components of a subjective and objective musculoskeletal health history utilizing critical thinking and therapeutic communication to support rapid focused assessment leading to accurate collaborative care.
- Describe age-related changes in the musculoskeletal system.
- Describe common musculoskeletal health problems.
- Describe the nursing process in which musculoskeletal problems may occur.
- Identify common musculoskeletal medications.

Section I. Overview of the Musculoskeletal System

Case Scenario: A 70-year-old client was admitted to the emergency department after a fall in her home. She is accompanied by her daughter. The client states that she was using a stepstool to reach for an item in her kitchen cabinet and slipped off the stool and fell. Her daughter states she was in the bedroom and came out after she heard her mother yell. She states she found her on the floor in the kitchen on her right side. She is alert and oriented x 3. She states her pain is a 7 out of 10 to her right hip. Denies any other pain. History reveals that the client has hypertension and cardiovascular disease. Medications include Lopressor 100 mg daily, Lasix 20 mg daily, and a daily multivitamin.

Vital signs: T: 98.8, P: 98, R: 28, BP: 166/88.

Orders: X-ray and CT scan to bilateral hips, CBC, serum electrolytes, pulse oximetry: 97%, U/A. PT, PTT.

Self Study Guide

Complete the following as you listen to the lecture and/or refer to your textbook.

Musculoskeletal System

Bones (Define Each Type)

Long Bones:

_____
_____
_____
_____

Short Bones:

_____
_____
_____
_____

Flat Bones:

_____
_____
_____
_____

Compact Bones:

_____
_____
_____
_____

Spongy Bones:

_____
_____
_____
_____

Hormonal Influences: How does each hormone influence growth and loss of bone?

Estrogen:

_____
_____
_____

Calcitonin:

_____
_____
_____

Parathyroid Hormone:

_____
_____
_____

Growth Hormone:

_____
_____
_____

Muscles (Define Each Type)

Skeletal:

_____
_____
_____
_____

Smooth:

_____
_____
_____

Cardiac:

_____
_____
_____
_____

Joints (Define Each Type)

Synovial:

_____
_____
_____
_____

Non-synovial:

_____
_____
_____
_____

What is the role of each?

Synovial Fluid:

_____
_____
_____
_____

Cartilage:

_____
_____
_____
_____

Bursa:

_____
_____
_____
_____

Describe the functional classification of joints

Synarthrosis:

_____

_____

_____

_____

Amphiarthrosis:

_____

_____

_____

_____

Diarthrosis:

_____

_____

_____

_____

Define each of these

Ligament:

_____

_____

_____

_____

Tendons:

_____

_____

_____

_____

Fascia:

_____

_____

_____

_____

Section I. Application Exercise 1

The client's labs and diagnostic test reveal a fracture to the right hip. She was taken to surgery and had a right hip arthroplasty. The procedure was uneventful, and the client is in the PACU. The client has an IV of D5W with 0.49 of normal saline infusing to left forearm, PCA pump with morphine sulfate at 1 mg/hr, and O_2 via nasal cannula at 2L. Dressing to right hip with Hemovac drain. She remains stable and is transferred to the unit.

The following orders are given: Clear liquid diet and advance as tolerated. Circulation, movement, sensation, and temperature checks q 2 hours; assess wound, wound drainage, and change dressing as needed with dry sterile dressing and document drainage from wound. Monitor PCA and up in chair this evening.

Prioritize what the nursing interventions would do in caring for the client.

Take vital signs	
Check dressing	
Assess for pain	
Get client up in chair	
Check CMST to right leg	

Assessment: Past Medical History, Present Illness

_____

_____

_____

_____

_____

_____

_____

Physical Assessment

Posture: Define the Following:

Lordosis:

_____

_____

Kyphosis:

_____

_____

Swayback:

_____

_____

Scoliosis:

_____

_____

Gait: Why is a person's gait so important in your assessment of mobility?

_____

_____

_____

_____

_____

_____

_____

_____

Joint Mobility (Define)

_____

_____

_____

_____

What is a goniometer?

_____

_____

Why is it used?

_____

_____

Sensation

How Does Sensation Affect Bone Function?

_____

_____

_____

_____

_____

_____

_____

Pulse Assessment

What Do Pulses Tell About Blood Flow?

_____

_____

_____

_____

_____

_____

_____

Muscle Tone and Strength:

_____

_____

_____

_____

_____

_____

_____

Section I. Application Exercise 2

It is the second day postop and the client has had her Hemovac removed. Dry sterile dressing is over right hip staples. The client's PCA pump and IV fluid have also been removed. Saline lock in place. Client has order for oral pain meds, stool softener prn, and continues her blood pressure medications. She has some bilateral crackles to lungs and nonproductive cough. She also complains of SOB while getting out of bed for her exercises.

Based on the above information, identify a primary diagnosis and prioritize the interventions for the client.

Primary Diagnosis		Interventions
		Notify physician
		Take vital signs
		Check O_2 saturation
		Increase fluids
		Have client use incentive spirometer

Diagnostic Tests

X-ray:

_____

_____

Nursing Care and/Client Preparation:

_____

_____

_____

_____

Computed Tomography:

_____

_____

Nursing Care and/Client Preparation:

_____

_____

_____

_____

Magnetic Resonance Imaging:

_____

_____

Nursing Care and/Client Preparation:

_____

_____

_____

_____

Arthrogram:

_____

_____

Nursing Care and/Client Preparation:

_____

_____

_____

_____

Bone Densities:

_____

_____

Nursing Care and/Client Preparation:

_____

_____

_____

_____

Bone Scan:

_____

_____

Nursing Care and/Client Preparation:

_____

_____

_____

_____

Electromyography:

_____

_____

Nursing Care and/Client Preparation:

_____

_____

_____

_____

Arthroscopic Examination:

_____

_____

Nursing Care and/Client Preparation:

_____

_____

_____

_____

Age-Related Changes

What changes occur with the following:

Bone Density:

_____
_____
_____
_____

Joint Cartilage:

_____
_____
_____
_____

Connective Tissue:

_____
_____
_____
_____

Muscle Fibers:

_____
_____
_____
_____

Dowager's Hump (Define):

_____
_____

Sarcopenia (Define):

_____
_____

Section I. Application Exercise 3

The client is stable and is preparing to be discharged. Develop a teaching plan for discharge for the client.

Teaching Plan

Medications	
Diet	
Exercise	
Home Management	
Pain Management	

Section II. Musculoskeletal Disorders

Case Scenario: A 10-year-old male is seen in the emergency department with increased difficulty walking. He is accompanied by his parents. They state that the client needs help to climb the stairs at home and seems to be weak. The client states he cannot participate in PE classes without getting tired. Assessment reveals muscle weakness in lower extremities, leg pain, and calf enlargement.

Vital signs: T: 98.8, P: 110, R: 12, BP: 96/58, pulse oximetry: 96%.

Labs ordered: Chest X-ray, ECG; lab studies: CK, LD, ALT, AST, lactic acid levels, serum creatinine.

Tidbit

The different types of muscular dystrophies affect over 50,000 people in the United States. The average lifespan of a person diagnosed with Duchenne muscular dystrophy is roughly 20 years. However, people diagnosed with Becker muscular dystrophy are said to have a normal life expectancy.

Muscular Dystrophies

Define:

_____
_____
_____
_____

Etiology/Pathophysiology:

_____
_____

_____
_____
_____
_____
_____
_____
_____
_____
_____

Manifestations:

_____
_____
_____
_____

Two Main Subgroups

Duchenne:

_____
_____
_____
_____

Becker:

_____
_____
_____
_____

Diagnostic Tests:

_____
_____
_____
_____

Section II. Application Exercise 1

Looking at the tests ordered for the client, determine the reason for each and its implication.

Creatine Kinase (CK):

_____
_____

Lactate Dehydrogenase (LD):

_____

_____

Alanine Aminotransferase (ALT):

_____

_____

Aspartate Aminotransferase (AST):

_____

_____

Medical Management:

_____

_____

_____

_____

_____

_____

_____

_____

Nursing Management:

_____

_____

_____

_____

_____

_____

_____

_____

Section II. Application Exercise 2

The labs indicate muscular dystrophy. The client is placed on corticosteroids and given ibuprofen for pain. Physical therapy has been ordered for the client and fall precautions are in place. Genetic counseling is also ordered for the parents.

Develop a **nursing care plan using the following diagnoses for muscular dystrophy.**

Nursing Diagnosis	Intervention	Rationale
Impaired physical mobility		
Risk for falls		
Risk for ineffective breathing pattern		
Risk for dysphagia		
Ineffective health maintenance		

Case Scenario: A 65-year-old female presents to the health care provider's office with complaints of difficulty walking. She states she has a family history of osteoporosis, so she states she makes sure she takes her calcium and vitamin supplements and tries to exercise 2–3 times a week. The client states she doesn't have any pain, but she is stiff as she walks, and this has limited her exercise. Assessment reveals a slumped posture, skin warm, dry. Turgor good. Lungs clear bilaterally.

Vital signs: T: 98.7, P: 88, R: 26, BP: 188/86, pulse oximetry: 99%.

Diagnostic tests ordered: DEXA scan, BMD, serum electrolytes, ESR.

Osteoporosis

Etiology/Pathophysiology:

_____

_____

_____

_____

Osteoclasts:

_____

_____

Osteoblasts:

_____

_____

Osteopenia:

_____

_____

_____

_____

Risk Factors

Primary List

Genetics:

_____

_____

_____

_____

Secondary List

Nutrition:

_____

_____

_____

_____

Lifestyle:

_____

_____

_____

_____

Manifestations:

_____

_____

_____

_____

Diagnostic Tests:

_____

_____

_____

_____

Section II. Application Exercise 3

Since the client is over the age of 65, the gold standard for assessing osteoporosis is a DEXA scan. Describe below the purpose of this test and what it reveals.

DEXA Scan:

_____

_____

_____

Medical Management:

_____

_____

_____

_____

_____

_____

_____

_____

Section II. Application Exercise 4

The client's BMD is −2.5. Physical therapy has been ordered for muscle-strengthening exercises and weight-bearing exercises. The patient also is continuing her calcium of 1200 mg and vitamin D 2000 IU per day. In addition, she has also been prescribed a bisphosphate (Boniva). Complete the chart below of the pharmacological interventions for osteoporosis.

Class	Dosage Schedule	Nursing Considerations	Mechanism of Action

Bisphosphates
    Alendronate (Fosamax)
    Ibandronate (Boniva)
    Risedronate (Actonel)
    Zoledronate (Reclast)			

Calcitonin Miacalcin/Fortical			

Estrogen Therapy
    Estrace
    Estraderm
    Premarin			

Estrogen Antagonist/ Agonist Raloxifene			

Parathyroid Hormone
    Forteo
    PTH			

Parathyroid Hormone Analog Abaloparatide			
Monoclonal Activity Denosumab			
Dual Acting Strontium Ranelate			

Nursing Management:

Assessment:

_____
_____
_____
_____
_____
_____

Diagnosis:

_____
_____
_____
_____

Planning/Interventions:

_____

_____

_____

_____

Evaluation:

_____

_____

_____

_____

Paget's Disease

Etiology/Pathophysiology:

_____

_____

_____

_____

_____

_____

_____

_____

> **Tidbit**
>
> Paget's disease does not always run in families; however, research suggests that a close relative of someone with Paget's disease is more likely to develop the disease than someone without an affected relative.

Section II. Application Exercise 5

Compare and contrast the role of osteoclasts with Paget's disease and osteoporosis.

Osteoclasts	
Osteoporosis	Paget's

Manifestations:

_____

_____

_____

_____

Diagnostic Tests:

_____
_____
_____
_____

Medical Management:

_____
_____
_____
_____

Surgical Management:

Osteotomy:

_____
_____
_____

Spinal Stabilization:

_____
_____
_____

Section II. Application Exercise 6

Develop a care plan for Paget's disease using the following diagnoses:

- Acute/Chronic Pain
- Impaired Physical Mobility
- Risk for Falls

Nursing Diagnosis	Client Goals	Interventions	Rationale
1. Acute/Chronic Pain			
2. Impaired Physical Mobility			
3. Risk for Falls			

Case Scenario: A 20-year-old male is seen in the emergency department with right hip pain and an unsteady gait. The client states he had minor trauma to the right hip 3 days ago after he was hit with a baseball during a game. The client states he has had a fever for 3 days and has been taking ibuprofen for pain for the last week. The client has limited ROM to right hip and cannot bear weight on the right leg. The client rates his pain an 8 out of 10.

Vital signs: T: 100.1, P: 96, R: 28, BP: 98/60, pulse oximetry: 97%.

Labs ordered: CBC, C-reactive protein, ESR, blood cultures, MRI of right hip.

Osteomyelitis

Etiology/Pathophysiology:

_____

_____

_____

_____

Three Categories

Acute Infection:

_____

_____

_____

_____

Subacute Infection:

_____

_____

_____

_____

Chronic Infection:

_____

_____

_____

_____

> **Tidbit**
> Osteomyelitis can affect both adults and children. In adults, osteomyelitis often affects the vertebrae and the pelvis. In children, osteomyelitis usually affects the adjacent ends of long bones.

Section II. Application Exercise 7

The client's MRI shows a lesion to the right femur. Blood studies and blood culture are positive *Staphylococcus aureus*. The following orders are given: IV infusion of Ceftazidime and oxacillin for 7 days, Tylenol 500 mg, oral q 4–6 hours as needed, thermal therapy q 4 hours. Gentle ROM exercises above and below affected site. High-protein diet. Prioritize the orders given for the client.

_____ ROM exercises

_____ Administer pain meds

_____ Assess client for vital signs and pain

_____ Assess IV site

_____ Infused IV antibiotics

_____ Thermal therapy

_____ Instruct on high-protein diet.

Manifestations:

_____
_____
_____
_____

Diagnostic Tests:

_____
_____
_____
_____

Medical Management:

_____
_____
_____
_____
_____
_____
_____
_____

Nursing Management:

Assessment:

_____
_____
_____
_____
_____
_____

Diagnosis:

_____
_____
_____
_____

Planning/Interventions:

_____
_____
_____
_____

Evaluation:

_____
_____
_____
_____

Section II. Application Exercise 8

The client completes the 7-day course of IV antibiotics. His pain is minimal, and he can do active ROM to affected extremity. He is being prepared for discharge and is sent home with oral antibiotics. Create a discharge teaching plan for the client.

| Pain Management |
| Oral Antibiotic |
| Diet Teaching |
| Activity |

Scoliosis

Etiology/Pathophysiology:

_____
_____
_____
_____

Manifestations:

_____
_____
_____
_____

Diagnostic Tests:

_____
_____
_____
_____

Medical Management:

_____
_____
_____
_____
_____
_____
_____

Nursing Management:

Assessment:

_____
_____
_____
_____
_____
_____

Diagnosis:

_____
_____
_____
_____

Planning/Interventions:

_____
_____
_____
_____

Evaluation:

_____
_____
_____
_____

Section II. Application Exercise 9

Using the word list, complete the concept map for scoliosis.

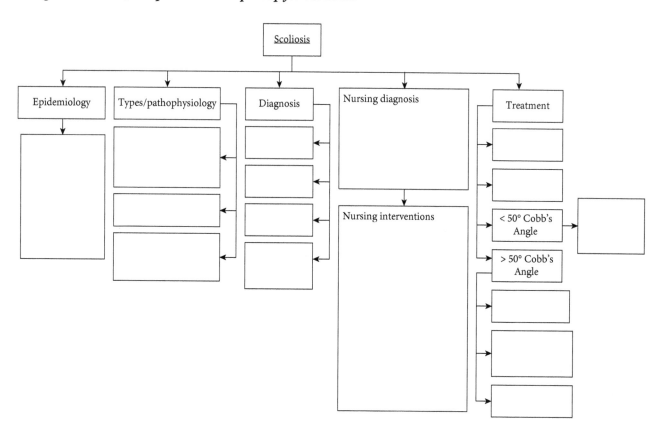

Word List for Scoliosis Concept Map

Idiopathic: unknown cause   Cobb angle

Nonsteroidal analgesia   Radiographic studies

Structural alteration noted by a curvature of the spine greater than 10°.

Risk factors: smoking, obesity, older age, heavy lifting, sedentary lifestyle

Congenital: asymmetry due to congenital anomaly
Neuromuscular: cerebral palsy, myelomeningocele, muscular dystrophy

Spinal instrumentation   Adams forward bending test

Scoliometer   Opioids

Thoracic-lumbar spinal orthotic (TLSO) Thermal, physical, occupational therapies

History and physical

Acute/chronic pain

Impaired physical mobility

Risk for falls

Risk for pathological fractures

Disturbed body image

Administered pain meds as ordered

Maintain orthotic device

Apply thermal therapy as ordered

Assist with ROM

Refer to PT, OT therapy

Instruct on managing TLSO brace

Instruct on maintaining a level of activity

Provide encouragement about body image and ways to cope

Case Scenario: Mrs. O'Reilly is a 78-year-old female who is seen in the health care provider's office with a history of osteoarthritis. She states her pain and stiffness have been increasing to her left hip and it is difficult to get up from a sitting position. The client is 5'4" and weighs 225 lbs. She lives alone and has been independent in a senior living village. She has a nurse who comes to her apartment twice a week for medication reminders. The client was put on a weight control diet, exercise modification, and given steroid injections to left hip in the past, but still no improvement of pain shown. The health care provider considers surgery.

Vital signs: T: 99.8, P: 96, R: 22, BP: 168/88, pulse oximetry: 98%.

Labs ordered: X-ray and MRI to left hip, CMP, CBC, PT/PTT, ECG.

Total Joint Replacement (TJR)

Etiology/Pathophysiology:

_____
_____
_____
_____

Tidbit

Total joint replacement has been around since the 1950s. The profile of the patients having hip surgery is changing from the elderly person with minimal needs to the young adult who wishes to have the maximum from their hip.

_____

_____

_____

_____

_____

_____

_____

_____

_____

Section II. Application Exercise 10

Match the indications for total joint replacement surgery with the diagnosis.

Indication	Diagnosis
Femoral head death due to alcohol or trauma; can be years after an episode	Developmental dysplasia, misalignment of femur and hip, Perthes disease
Degeneration of articular cartilage and bony cyst formation	Bony ankylosis if hip joint
Previous childhood hip diseases	Rheumatoid arthritis
Intracapsular fractured neck of femur	Abnormal wearing away of the joint surfaces due to injury or surgery
Previous injury or surgery to joint	Done for patient with underlying osteoarthritis in fractured hip; femoral head replaced
Ankylosis spondylitis	Avascular necrosis of the femoral head (THR)
Bony erosion and destruction of articular cartilage	Osteoarthritis

Manifestations:

_____

_____

_____

_____

Diagnostic Tests:

_____

_____

_____

_____

Section II. Application Exercise 11

X-rays and MRI show muscle atrophy tissue destruction of left hip. Hgb and HCT normal. ECG normal, coagulation studies within normal limits. Client is a good candidate for surgery and will have a left total hip arthroplasty. Develop a pre- and postop teaching plan for the client.

Preoperative	Postoperative
Education about the procedure

Vital signs:

Labs:

Pain Management: | Vital signs:

Medication Management:

Diet:

Wound assessment:

Neuro checks:

Activity: |

Nursing Management:

Assessment:

_____
_____
_____
_____
_____
_____

Diagnosis:

_____
_____
_____
_____

Planning/Interventions:

_____
_____
_____
_____

Evaluation:

_____
_____
_____
_____

Case Scenario: Jimmy, a 14-year-old boy, was brought into the emergency department by his mother. Jimmy was skateboarding at the park and fell off his skateboard. The client comes in with edema and pain to right ankle and an abrasion to his right knee. The client states, "I think I broke my ankle." He rates his pain as a 6 out of 10. There is no significant history for the client. Site is warm and is sensitive to touch. The health care provider orders an X-ray of the affected extremity.

   Vitals: T: 99, P: 94, R: 16, BP: 100/70, pulse oximetry: 99%.

Strains and Sprains

Etiology/Pathophysiology:

_____
_____
_____

Tidbit

Strains and sprains affect all ages and are the most prevalent type of musculoskeletal injuries in the United States.

Section II. Application Exercise 12

Create a chart to differentiate between the different types of strains and sprains.

	Severity	Manifestations
Strains		
Sprains		

Diagnostic Tests:

_____
_____
_____
_____

Medical Management:

_____
_____
_____
_____

Section II. Application Exercise 13

The client's X-rays show a first-degree sprain to right ankle. Treatment will include <u>RICE</u>. Discuss what this acronym means in terms of treatment of the sprain and the rationale for each.

R: _____

I: _____

C: _____

E: _____

Nursing Management:

_____
_____
_____
_____

Section II. Application Exercise 14

Develop a care plan using the following nursing diagnoses for sprains and strains:

Impaired physical mobility, acute pain, impaired tissue perfusion, knowledge deficit.

Assessment:

_____
_____
_____
_____
_____

Diagnosis:

_____
_____
_____
_____

Planning/Interventions:

_____
_____
_____
_____

Evaluation:

_____
_____
_____
_____

Case Scenario: A 67-year-old male is seen in the emergency department after a fall from his wheelchair at the retirement home. The client is not able to move his left arm and states he fell "right on top of it." Rates pain as a 9 out of 10. Left arm is immobile and is in a flexed position. Client has a history of hypertension and COPD. He is on O_2 at 3l via nasal cannula, is alert and oriented. The health care provider has ordered an X-ray to left arm.

Vital signs: T: 99.4, P: 96, R: 24, BP: 165/86.

Fractures

Etiology/Pathophysiology:

Define:

_____
_____
_____
_____

Types

Complete:

_____
_____

Incomplete:

_____
_____

Closed or Simple:

_____
_____

Open or Compound:

_____
_____

Grade I:

_____
_____

Grade II:

_____
_____

Grade III:

Patterns of Fractures

Avulsion:

_____

_____

Compression:

_____

_____

Comminuted

Displaced:

_____

_____

Depressed:

_____

_____

Greenstick:

_____

_____

Spiral:

_____

_____

Nondisplaced:

_____

_____

Oblique:

_____

_____

Impacted:

_____

_____

Diagnostic Tests:

_____

_____

_____

_____

Section II. Application Exercise 15

The client's X-rays reveal a closed, nondisplaced fracture to left elbow. Do you think a surgical or nonsurgical management plan should be implemented for the client? Why? Discuss each type of surgical and nonsurgical management.

Nonsurgical Management

_____

_____

_____

_____

_____

_____

_____

_____

_____

Surgical Management

_____

_____

_____

_____

_____

_____

_____

Traction

Define:

_____

_____

_____

Skeletal:

_____

_____

_____

_____

Skin:

_____

_____

_____

_____

Complications

Compartment Syndrome:

_____

_____

_____

_____

Neurovascular Compromise:

_____

_____

_____

_____

VTE:

_____

_____

_____

_____

Fat Embolism:

_____

_____

_____

_____

Rhabdomyolysis:

_____
_____
_____
_____

Hypovolemia:

_____
_____
_____
_____

Malunion/Nonunion:

_____
_____
_____
_____

Infection:

_____
_____
_____
_____

Section II. Application Exercise 16

The client has a cast applied to the left arm. The nurse must do teaching on cast care. Discuss what you will teach the client about proper care of the cast.

	Cast Care
Proper Care:	
Things to Avoid:	

Nursing Management:

Assessment:

_____
_____
_____
_____
_____
_____

Diagnosis:

_____
_____
_____
_____

Planning/Interventions:

_____
_____
_____
_____

Evaluation:

_____
_____
_____
_____

Amputations

Etiology/Pathophysiology:

Define:

_____
_____
_____
_____

Traumatic Amputations:

_____
_____
_____
_____

Elective Amputations:

_____
_____
_____
_____

> **Tidbit**
>
> Most amputations are performed because of cardiovascular disease, diabetes, or other health conditions. The word *prosthesis* means "addition" in Greek.

Complications

Phantom Limb Pain:

_____

_____

_____

_____

_____

Section II. Application Exercise 17

The following diagnoses apply to the client with phantom limb pain: Acute/chronic pain, impaired skin integrity, grieving, ineffective coping, ineffective tissue perfusion.

Choose two of the above diagnoses as a priority and develop a care plan for each.

Nursing Diagnosis	Patient Outcomes	Nursing Interventions/ Rationale	Evaluation
1.			
2.			

Critical Thinking Questions

1. Which information will the nurse teach seniors at a community recreation center about ways to prevent fractures?

    a. Tack down scatter rugs in the home.

    b. Expect most falls to happen outside the home.

    c. Buy shoes that provide good support and are comfortable to wear.

    d. Get instruction in range-of-motion exercises from a physical therapist.

2. In which order will the nurse take these actions when caring for a patient in the emergency department with a right leg fracture after a motor vehicle crash? (*Put in priority number order.*)

    a. Obtain X-rays.   _____

    b. Check pedal pulses.   _____

    c. Assess lung sounds.   _____

    d. Take blood pressure.   _____

    e. Apply splint to the leg.   _____

    f. Administer tetanus prophylaxis.   _____

3. When caring for a patient who is using Buck's traction after a hip fracture, which action can the nurse delegate to unlicensed assistive personnel (UAP)?

    a. Remove and reapply traction periodically.

    b. Ensure the weight for the traction is hanging freely.

    c. Monitor the skin under the traction boot for redness.

    d. Check for intact sensation and movement in the affected leg.

4. Before assisting a patient with ambulation 2 days after total hip arthroplasty, which action is **most** important for the nurse to take?

    a. Observe output from the surgical drain.

    b. Administer prescribed pain medication.

    c. Instruct the patient about benefits of early ambulation.

    d. Change the dressing and document the wound appearance.

Chapter 13

Sensory Alterations

Introduction

This chapter will examine sensory alterations and the disease processes related to them.

T HE VISUAL AND auditory systems are part of the sensory system. The eyes take in light, convert it to electrical signals, and then send it to the brain along the optic nerve, where it is processed in order to make decisions. The inner surface of the eye, the retina, is the light-sensitive area and it is like a camera. Rods and cones detect color and light. The lens helps with focus, while the cornea is the transparent covering of the iris and pupil; along with the lens, it refracts light so it can be projected onto the retina. The pupil is the central part of the eye and the iris, which can be different colors, controls the size of the pupil.

The ears not only assist in hearing but also with balance. The external ear, or the pinna, works like a megaphone. Sound travels through the external ear to the auditory canal to the tympanic membrane, or eardrum. The tympanic membrane is filled with air and mucosa and the auditory ossicles, which are the bones of the ear (malleus, incus, and stapes). As the bones vibrate, they send this vibration to the inner ear where the cochlea, which is a fluid-filled, spiral structure, lies. It is here that tiny hair cells turn the vibrations into electrical impulses that are carried to the brain by sensory nerves. The Eustachian tube is in the middle ear and assists with equalizing pressure to help with balance. The vestibular complex is in the inner ear. It has receptors that regulate equilibrium. It is connected to the vestibulocochlear nerve that carries sound and equilibrium information to the brain.

There are many disorders that affect the function of the eyes and ears. It is important to examine and understand the changes that occur to these organs and the disease processes associated with them.

Learning Objectives of This Chapter

Upon completion of this chapter, the student should be able to:

- Discuss the pathophysiology and clinical manifestations of imbalance of visual and auditory problems.
- Identify important components of a subjective and objective visual and auditory health history utilizing critical thinking and therapeutic communication to support rapid focused assessment leading to accurate collaborative care.

- Describe age-related changes in the visual and auditory systems.
- Describe common visual and auditory health problems.
- Describe the nursing process in which visual and auditory problems may occur.
- Identify common visual and auditory medications.

Section I. Extraocular Disorders

Case Scenario: A 44-year-old female is seen in the optometrist's office with complaints of changes to her vision. She states she is an editor at a well-known publishing company and is responsible for a large department. She states, "I always have had perfect vision and pride myself on that. I have a sister who is nearsighted and one who is farsighted, but I have always had 20/20 vision. Now it is difficult to see up close as I read." The health care provider conducts vision testing on the client.

Self Study Guide

Complete the following as you listen to the lecture and/or refer to your textbook.

Tidbit
Age-related eye diseases are the leading cause of blindness and decreased vision in the United States. Approximately 11 million Americans aged 12 years and older could improve their vision through proper refractive correction.

Vision Testing

Purpose:

_____
_____
_____
_____

Snellen Chart:

_____
_____
_____
_____

Jaeger Card:

_____
_____
_____
_____

Ishihara Test:

_____
_____
_____

Confrontation Test:

_____

_____

_____

_____

Corneal Light Reflex:

_____

_____

_____

_____

Six Cardinal Positions of Gaze:

_____

_____

_____

_____

Section I. Application Exercise 1

There are several diagnostic tests that are done to gather information to determine treatment for ocular disorders. Match the different diagnostic tests with their purpose.

Radioisotope Scanning	Provides detailed images about internal eye circulation by injecting an IV dye.
Slit-lamp Testing	Grid used to determine macular degeneration.
Corneal Staining Test	Small amounts of radioactive substances injected into body to identify tumors and ocular melanomas.
Fluorescein Angiography	High-intensity light magnification to look for cataracts, macular degeneration, glaucoma, or conjunctivitis in the back of the eye.
Computed Tomography	Use of high-frequency soundwaves to produce images of soft tissue.
Ultrasonography	Scans to diagnose diseases of blood vessels, eye muscles, optic nerve; done with or without contrast.
Intraocular Testing	Gives detailed image of eye structures.
Magnetic Resonance Imaging	Tonometer used to measure eyeball pressure.
Amsler Grid Test	Orange dye placed in eye to detect scratches or foreign bodies on the cornea.

Age-related Changes

_____

_____

_____

_____

_____
_____
_____

Refraction Errors

Refraction

Define:

_____
_____
_____
_____

Section I. Application Exercise 2

The client's visual exam reveals that she has presbyopia. Differentiate between the different types of refractive errors and their meaning and risk factors.

Refractive Disorder	Meaning	Risk Factors
Hyperopia		
Myopia		
Astigmatism		
Presbyopia		

Surgical Management:

_____
_____
_____
_____

Section I. Application Exercise 3

The health care provider reviews the medical and surgical treatments for the client's presbyopia. The client has expressed that she would like to know more about the different modalities for her condition. For each type of condition, state the types of lenses used and surgical treatments.

Refractive Disorder	Lens	Treatment
Hyperopia		
Myopia		
Astigmatism		
Presbyopia		

Nursing Interventions and Patient Teaching:

_____
_____
_____
_____
_____
_____
_____
_____

Section I. Application Exercise 4

The client has decided to use corrective lenses for her presbyopia. Develop a teaching plan for the client.

Importance of Wearing Eyeglasses or Contact Lenses:

_____
_____
_____
_____

Follow-up Eye Care:

_____
_____
_____

Reporting Eye Problems:

_____
_____
_____

Section II. Infectious Eye Disorders

Case Scenario: A 20-year-old female presents to her health provider's office with complaints of irritation to right eye. The eye is red, and purulent drainage is noted at the inner canthus of the eye. She states it feels like sand is in her eye She is a preschool teacher and states that she noticed the irritation yesterday and woke up with purulent drainage on her pillow and difficulty opening her right eye. Upon assessment, the nurse finds that the client's sclera is pinkish and inflamed.

Vital signs: T: 99.2, P: 86, R: 22, BP: 146/76, pulse oximetry: 98%.

Conjunctivitis (Pink Eye)

Define:

_____
_____
_____

Acute Bacterial Conjunctivitis/Manifestations:

_____
_____
_____

Viral Conjunctivitis/Manifestations:

_____
_____
_____

Allergic Conjunctivitis/Manifestations:

_____
_____
_____

Chlamydial Conjunctivitis/Manifestations:

_____
_____
_____

Mechanical Conjunctivitis/Manifestations:

_____
_____
_____

> *Tidbit*
>
> One of the most common and most harmful misconceptions about pink eye is that there's only one highly contagious type. Pink eye has numerous causes, including allergies, exposure to chemical fumes, advanced dry eye, and infections.

Toxic Conjunctivitis/Manifestations:

_____
_____
_____

Traumatic Conjunctivitis/Manifestations:

_____
_____
_____

Section II. Application Exercise

The client has been diagnosed with bacterial conjunctivitis. Prioritize the following nursing actions that the nurse will implement for the client.

_____	Referral to an eye care specialist for any other eye problems
_____	Teach good hand hygiene
_____	Teach transmission prevention at home
_____	Administer prescribed medications
_____	Provide comfort measures
_____	Discuss follow-up care

Treatment Plan for the Types of Conjunctivitis

Acute Bacterial Conjunctivitis:

_____
_____
_____

Viral Conjunctivitis:

_____
_____
_____

Allergic Conjunctivitis:

_____
_____
_____

Chlamydial Conjunctivitis:

_____
_____
_____

Mechanical Conjunctivitis:

_____
_____
_____

Toxic Conjunctivitis:

_____
_____
_____

Traumatic Conjunctivitis:

_____
_____
_____

Infections of the External Eye

Hordeolum (Stye):

_____
_____
_____
_____
_____
_____

Chalazion:

_____
_____
_____
_____
_____
_____

Blepharitis:

_____
_____
_____
_____
_____
_____
_____

Corneal Disorders

Abrasion:

_____
_____
_____

Foreign Bodies:

_____
_____
_____

Viral:

_____
_____
_____

Bacterial:

_____
_____
_____

Spontaneous Defects

Eye Abrasions:

_____
_____
_____

Trauma:

_____
_____
_____

Dry Eyes:

_____
_____
_____

Section III. Ocular Disorders

Case Scenario: Mr. Thomas, a 76-year-old male, has been referred to the ophthalmologist's office by his primary care provider. The client has a history of diabetes mellitus and hypertension. The client states he manages his diabetes with daily insulin injections and checks his blood sugars 3 times a day. He takes amlodipine for his blood pressure. The client states that his vision is blurry and distorted and he cannot see very well at night. The ophthalmologist conducts a slit lamp exam to look at the back of the eye.

Cataracts

Define:

_____
_____
_____
_____
_____
_____

Clinical Manifestations:

_____
_____
_____
_____
_____

Assessment:

_____
_____

Tidbit

According to the World Health Organization, cataracts cause a third of worldwide blindness, affecting approximately 65.2 million people. Cataracts additionally cause moderate to severe vision loss to 52.6 million individuals, 99% of whom live in developing countries.

_____
_____
_____
_____

Diagnostic Test:

_____
_____
_____
_____
_____
_____

Surgical Management:

_____
_____
_____
_____
_____
_____

Section III. Application Exercise 1

The slit lamp exam reveals an opaqueness in the back of the eye. A diagnosis of cataracts is confirmed. The client has an extracapsular cataract extraction procedure done. The nurse is assigned to do postop care and teaching. Discuss what is to be taught and the rationale for the following care for the client.

Postop Care and Teaching	Rationale
Eye Care	
Positioning	
Safety	
Stool Softeners	
Diet	
Follow-up Care	

Case Scenario: A 39-year-old client is seen in the ophthalmologist's office with complaints of deteriorating vision to both eyes for the last 2 years. She states this change has been gradual but has been more bothersome to her lately. The client states she cannot see things that are not directly in front of her. The client states she has headaches at times and complains of nausea but no vomiting. Visual acuity exam and tonometer exam done.

Glaucoma

Define:

_____
_____
_____

Intraocular Pressure (IOP):

_____
_____
_____

Clinical Manifestations

Primary Open Angle Glaucoma:

_____
_____
_____

Narrow-Angle Glaucoma:

_____
_____
_____

Normal Tension Glaucoma:

_____
_____
_____

Secondary Glaucoma:

_____
_____
_____

Pediatric Glaucoma:

_____
_____
_____

Assessment:

_____
_____
_____
_____
_____
_____

Diagnostic Tests:

_____
_____
_____
_____
_____

Section III. Application Exercise 2

The tonometer reading reflects an IOP of 26. Opthalmoscope reveals bulging vessels in external eye. Client has difficulty with vision eye exam, stating the letters look "foggy" on the Snellen chart. A diagnosis of primary open-angle glaucoma is made. The client is prescribed Timoptic drops to both eyes. The client asks what this medication does. Fill in the chart below to describe the purpose of each type of medication to treat glaucoma.

Medication	Purpose/Effect
Prostaglandin-type Medications • Bimatoprost (Lumigan) • Latanoprost (Xalatan)	
Epinephrine Compounds • Dipivefrin (Propine)	
Carbon Anhydrase Inhibitors • Brinzolamide (Azopt) • Dorzolamide (Trusopt)	
Beta-blocker Medications • Timolol (Betimol, Timoptic) • Betazolol (Betoptic) • Metipranolol (OptiPranolol)	
Alpha Antagonist • Brimonidine (Alphagan) • Apraclonidine (Iopidine)	
Miotic/Cholinergic Medications • Carbachol (Isopto Carbachol) • Pilocarpine (Isopto Carpine)	

Surgical Management:

Laser Trabeculoplasty:

_____
_____
_____

Trabeculectomy:

_____
_____
_____

Drainage Implants:

_____
_____
_____

Section III. Application Exercise 3

The client is being sent home with her eye medication. Before she leaves, the health care provider wants the nurse to teach eye drop installation. Prioritize the steps of the teaching plan on self-administration of eye drops.

Pull lower eye lid downward.   _____

Gently squeeze the bottle to allow drop to fall into
conjunctival sac. Do not contaminate dropper by   _____
touching the eye.

Another eye drop can be given after 3–5 minutes   _____
after first drop to allow for absorption.

Wash hands, apply gloves.   _____

Invert medication bottle.   _____

Tilt head back with eye open and looking upward.   _____

Check label for correct medication, dose, and   _____
number of drops.

Close eyes.   _____

Apply gentle pressure using tissue on the inner   _____
eye (nasolacrimal duct) for 30 seconds to decrease
absorption into the body.

Strabismus

Define:

_____
_____
_____

Esotropia: _____

Exotropia _____

Hypertropia: _____

Hypotropia:

_____
_____
_____
_____

Case Scenario: Mrs. Donner, a 50-year-old female, was seen in the optometrist's office for her scheduled exam. She states she has suddenly lost her vison to her right eye. She states she cannot stand bright lights and sees things "floating" at times or like there is something always in her eye like a veil. The client denies pain or headaches. The slit lamp exam reveals that the cornea of the right eye is red and is more dilated than the left eye.

Retinal Detachment

Define:

_____
_____
_____

Types

Rhegmatogenous:

_____
_____
_____

Tractional:

_____
_____
_____

Exudative:

_____
_____
_____

Tidbit

A retinal detachment can occur at any age, but it is more common in people over age 40. It affects men more than women, and Whites more than African Americans.

Section III. Application Exercise 4

The client has been diagnosed with rhegmatogenous retinal detachment and is scheduled for laser photoco-agulation surgery. Create a preop and postop care plan for the client.

Preop Teaching/Instructions	Interventions	Rationale
1. Teaching about procedure		
2. Wash face with antibacterial solution		
3. Cover both eyes		
4. Encourage quiet and restful environment		
5. Administer preop medications		

Postop Teaching/Care	Interventions	Rationale
1. Eye patch care		
2. Eye drop administration		
3. Signs/symptoms to report		
4. Position and position changes		
5. Follow-up care		

One of Five Procedures May be Performed

1. Laser Photocoagulation:

_____
_____
_____
_____
_____
_____
_____

2. Cryotherapy:

_____
_____
_____
_____
_____
_____
_____

3. Electrodiathermy:

_____
_____
_____
_____
_____
_____
_____

4. Scleral Buckling:

_____
_____
_____
_____
_____
_____
_____

5. Pneumatic (Pertaining to Air or Gas) Retinopexy:

_____
_____

_____

_____

_____

_____

_____

Case Scenario: A 67-year-old female is seen by her optometrist for her annual exam. She states she has noticed a change in her vision since her last visit. She states she did not think it was a big deal and thought it was because her blood pressure was elevated. The client complains of blurred spots in the center of her vision but denies pain. The client's history reveals hypertension, smoking x 30+ years. The client is overweight and states she has a very stressful job as a hospital administrator.

Age-Related Macular Degeneration (ARMD)

Define:

_____

_____

_____

Two Types

Wet Macular Degeneration:

_____

_____

_____

Dry Macular Degeneration:

_____

_____

_____

> *Tidbit*
>
> Macular degeneration is the leading cause of vision loss, affecting more than 10 million Americans—more than cataracts and glaucoma combined. At present, macular degeneration is considered an incurable eye disease.

Section III. Application Exercise 5

List the modifiable and nonmodifiable risk factors for macular degeneration. What risk factors does the client have?

Modifiable	Nonmodifiable

Clinical Manifestations:

_____
_____
_____
_____
_____
_____
_____
_____

Assessment:

_____
_____
_____
_____
_____
_____

Diagnostic Tests

Tonometry:

_____
_____
_____

Amsler Grid:

_____
_____
_____

Section III. Application Exercise 6

The optometrist conducts a comprehensive exam on the client, including a tonometry and Amsler grid exam. Diagnosis of intermediate dry macular degeneration. The client is given nutritional information as treatment for her diagnosis. Discuss the nutritional recommendations for dry macular degeneration.

_____
_____
_____
_____
_____
_____

Medical Management

Wet Macular Degeneration

Photodynamic Therapy:

_____

_____

_____

_____

Anti-vascular Endothelial Growth Factor Therapy:

_____

_____

_____

_____

Section III. Application Exercise 7

Create a concept map for care of the client with macular degeneration.

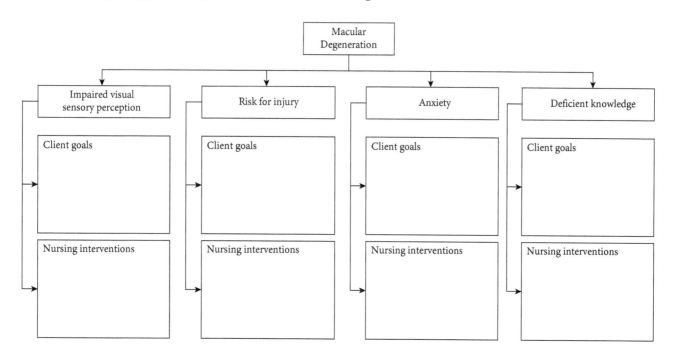

Eye Trauma

_____

_____

_____

_____

Risk Factors:

_____
_____
_____
_____

Manifestations:

_____
_____
_____
_____

Types and Treatment

Blunt Trauma:

_____
_____
_____
_____

Penetrating Eye Trauma:

_____
_____
_____
_____

Hyphema:

_____
_____
_____
_____

Globe Rupture:

_____
_____
_____
_____

Periorbital Wound:

_____

_____

_____

_____

Subconjunctival Hemorrhage:

_____

_____

_____

_____

Critical Thinking Questions

1. What should the nurse teach all patients with conjunctival infections to use?

    a. Artificial tears to moisten and soothe eyes.

    b. Dark glasses to prevent the discomfort of photophobia.

    c. Iced moist compresses to the eyes to promote comfort and healing.

    d. Frequent and thorough hand washing to avoid spreading the infection.

2. What nursing action is most important for the patient with age-related macular dry degeneration (AMD)?

    a. Teach the patient how to use topical eye drops for treatment of AMD.

    b. Emphasize the use of vision enhancement techniques to improve what vision is present.

    c. Encourage the patient to undergo laser treatment to slow deposit of cellular debris.

    d. Explain that nothing can be done to save the patient's vision because there is no treatment for AMD.

3. Which characteristics of glaucoma are associated with only acute primary angle-closure (PACG)? (*Select all that apply.*)

    a. Caused by lens blocking papillary opening.

    b. Treated with trabeculoplasty or trabeculectomy.

    c. Causes a loss of central vision with corneal edema.

    d. Treated with B-adrenergic blockers such as betaxolol (Betopic).

    e. Causes sudden, severe eye pain associated with nausea and vomiting.

    f. Treated with hyperosmotic oral and IV fluids to lower intraocular pressure.

4. Myopia is present in 25% of Americans. Which characteristics are associated with myopia? (*Select all that apply.*)

   a. Excessive light refraction

   b. Abnormally short eyeball

   c. Unequal corneal curvature

   d. Corrected with concave lens

   e. Image focused in front of retina

Chapter 14

Neurological Alterations

Introduction

This chapter will examine neurological alterations and the disease processes related to them.

T HE NERVOUS SYSTEM is a highly complex and very organized system in the body. Its role is to receive information via the nerves from sensory organs and transmit the information through the spinal cord up to the brain where the information is processed and sent back out to the body. This function controls the body's daily functions, from movement to the dilation of blood vessels. The nervous system consists of the central nervous system (CNS) and the peripheral nervous system (PNS). The excitatory or inhibitory stimulation of the neurotransmitters regulates the activity of muscles and glands. Neurotransmitters travel across synapses, spaces between neurons or between neurons and other body tissues and cells. The means of traveling for the neurologic activity is made possible by the spinal cord. Sensory and motor information travels up and down the spinal cord to and from the brain. Any interruption in this process along any part of the CNS or PNS can have devastating effects on the body.

Learning Objectives of This Chapter

Upon completion of this chapter, the student should be able to:

- Discuss the pathophysiology and clinical manifestations of imbalance of neurologic problems.
- Identify important components of a subjective and objective neurological health history utilizing critical thinking.
- Describe age-related changes in the neurological system.
- Describe common neurological health problems.
- Describe the nursing process in which neurological problems may occur.
- Identify common neurological medications.

Section I. Brain Disorders

Self Study Guide

Complete the following as you listen to the lecture and/or refer to your textbook.

Case Scenario: Carol, a 26-year-old soccer player, was involved in a head-on collision during a soccer game. She is complaining of a headache and some amnesia. Her coach brought her into the emergency department.

Vital signs: T: 98.2, R: 22, P: 96, BP: 126/76.

A neurological assessment and a CT scan of the head is performed.

Traumatic Brain Injury

Define:

_____

_____

_____

_____

Pathophysiology

Types of Head Injury

Scalp Laceration (Focal Injury):

_____

_____

_____

Contusion (Focal Injury):

Skull Fracture:

_____

_____

_____

Concussion (Diffuse Injury):

_____

_____

_____

> **Tidbit**
>
> Traumatic brain injury (TBI) is a leading cause of cognitive and brain problems occurring in millions of Americans every year. The CDC estimates that around 30% of all injury deaths are attributed to TBI.

Diffuse Axonal Injury:

_____
_____
_____

Diagnostic Tests:

_____
_____
_____
_____

Surgical Management:

_____
_____
_____
_____

Complications

Epidural Hematoma:

_____
_____
_____

Subdural Hematoma:

Acute:

_____
_____

Subacute:

_____
_____

Chronic:

_____
_____

Intracerebral Hematoma:

_____

_____

_____

Syndrome of Inappropriate Antidiuretic Hormone (SIADH):

_____

_____

_____

Diabetes Insipidus (DI):

_____

_____

_____

Section I. Application Exercise 1

The client is diagnosed with a minor concussion. The following orders have been given by the health care provider:

- Limit physical or any cognitive activities.
- No contact sports for the next 2 weeks until your follow-up with your health care provider.
- Tylenol 325 mg, 2 tabs q 4 hrs. prn.
- Do not stay home alone for the next 48 hrs.

The client and her coach need teaching on the client's condition. Prioritize the nurse's discharge teaching plan using the orders above.

Discharge Teaching	Rationale

Nursing Management

Assessment:

_____
_____
_____
_____

Diagnosis:

_____
_____
_____
_____

Interventions:

_____
_____
_____
_____

Intracranial Pressure

Define:

_____
_____
_____
_____

Monroe-Kellie Hypothesis:

_____
_____
_____
_____

Pathophysiology and Etiology:

_____
_____
_____
_____
_____

> *Tidbit*
>
> Increased intracranial pressure is a potential life-threatening event and involves the brain tissue, blood, and cerebrospinal fluid.

Section I. Application Exercise 2

The nurse assesses the client's level of consciousness and finds an 11 out of 15. What does this mean for the client?

_____

_____

Complete the responses and numbers for the Glasgow coma scale.

	NUMBER	MEANING
BEST EYE OPENING		
BEST MOTOR REPSONSE		
BEST VERBAL RESPONSE		

Signs and Symptoms

Early:

_____

_____

_____

_____

Late:

_____

_____

_____

_____

Cushing Triad

Define:

1. _____

2. _____

3. _____

Cheyne-Stokes Respiration:

_____

_____

_____

Abnormal Posturing

Decorticate:

_____

_____

_____

Decerebrate:

_____

_____

_____

Section I. Application Exercise 3

The health care provider conducts a neurological assessment, which reveals pupil irregularity. The client is becoming increasingly lethargic and had an episode of vomiting. CT and MRI scan done. The client is diagnosed with a concussion with increased intracranial pressure.

The following diagnoses apply to the client:

Ineffective cerebral tissue perfusion, ineffective breathing pattern, ineffective airway clearance, fluid volume deficit, disturbed thought process.

Select two priority diagnoses and create a care plan for the client.

Nursing Diagnosis	Intervention	Rationale

Medical Treatment:

What Is the Purpose of Mannitol for the ICP Client?

_____
_____
_____

Other Medications Used for ICP:

_____
_____
_____
_____

Nursing Considerations

Optimal Position for Client:

_____

Why?

_____
_____
_____
_____
_____

Case Scenario: Mr. Jones, 45 years old, has been seen by the health care provider due to headaches. He states he has been under a lot of stress from his job and because he is going through a divorce. He states the current management of his headaches using Tylenol are not working as the headaches come and go. The pain is described by the client as pressure to the frontal part of the head and neck. The client also states that he awakens with headaches at times. He states that he has not tried anything else for his pain. The client states the pain usually occurs several times a week, and this has been going on for the last few months.

Vital signs: T: 98.7, P: 96, R: 24, BP: 168/88.

Headaches

Types of Headaches

Define and Differentiate:

Migraine:

_____

_____

_____

> *Tidbit*
>
> Headaches are the most common pain experienced by people. There are several different types of headaches, and each type affects people in different ways.

Cluster:

_____

_____

_____

Tension:

_____

_____

_____

Section I. Application Exercise 4

Based on the physical exam and history, the health care provider has determined that the client is suffering from tension headaches. The health care provider has given the following orders:

- Ibuprofen 400 mg qid prn
- Amlodipine 5 mg qd
- Paxil 20 mg qd
- Instruct client on triggers that cause headaches
- Develop a priority nursing diagnosis and prioritize the interventions below

Priority Nursing Diagnosis

Administer prescribed meds   _____

Assess pain level   _____

Instruct on new medication regimen   _____

Encourage verbalization of feelings   _____

Discuss stressors that may trigger headaches   _____

Case Scenario: Ms. Kaplan, 25 years old, was brought into the emergency department by her mother. Her mother states that the client was cooking dinner and passed out for a few seconds and fell down. When the client regained consciousness, she did not remember the incident. Her mother states that their family has a history of seizures. Several tests were run, including an MRI, CT scan, and an EEG. Labs also drawn include CBC, serum glucose, and UA for drug screen.

Vital signs: T: 98.8, P: 82, R: 22, BP: 136/84.

Seizure Disorders

Classify Types

Focal Onset:

_____
_____
_____
_____

Generalized Onset:

_____
_____
_____
_____

Unknown Onset:

_____
_____
_____
_____

Manifestations

Preictal Phase:

_____
_____
_____
_____

Postictal Phase:

_____

_____

_____

_____

Diagnostic Tests:

_____

_____

_____

_____

Section I. Application Exercise 5

The client is admitted to the neurological unit. UA drug screen is negative. Other diagnostic data suggest seizure disorder. The nurse assigned the client is given the following orders:

- Vital signs and neuro checks q 4 hours
- Implement seizure precautions
- Bedrest
- Soft diet

Prioritize the nursing care and rationale for the client as she is admitted to the unit.

Priority   Rationale

_____ Implement seizure precautions

_____ Do admission assessment   _____

_____ Obtain vital signs

_____ Assess neurological status   _____

_____ Orientate the client to the room

_____ Document assessment   _____

_____ Inform health care provider of any relevant findings _____

Medications

Carbamazepine (Tegretol)

Class:

_____

_____

Used for Seizure Type:

_____

_____

Nursing Care:

_____

_____

Clonazepam (Klonopin)

Class:

_____

_____

Used for Seizure Type:

_____

_____

Nursing Care:

_____

_____

Gabapentin (Neurontin)

Class:

_____

_____

Used for Seizure Type:

_____

_____

Nursing Care:

_____

_____

Lamotrigine (Lamictal)

Class:

_____

_____

Used for Seizure Type:

_____

_____

Nursing Care:

_____

_____

Levetiracetam (Keppra)

Class:

_____

_____

Used for Seizure Type:

_____

_____

Nursing Care:

_____

_____

Phenobarbital (Luminal)

Class:

_____

_____

Used for Seizure Type:

_____

_____

Nursing Care:

_____

_____

Phenytoin (Dilantin)

Class:

_____

_____

Used for Seizure Type:

_____

_____

Nursing Care:

_____

_____

Pregabalin (Lyrica)

Class:

_____

_____

Used for Seizure Type:

_____

_____

Nursing Care:

_____

_____

Topiramate (Topamax)

Class:

_____

_____

Used for Seizure Type:

_____

_____

Nursing Care:

_____

_____

Valproate Acid (Depakote)

Class:

_____

_____

Used for Seizure Type:

_____

_____

Nursing Care:

_____

_____

Section I. Application Exercise 6

The heath care provider has prescribed Dilantin for the client. The client and her mother verbalize that even though they have a history of seizures in the family, they don't talk about it. They verbalize their confusion on how to manage the disorder.

Create a concept map for care of the client with seizure disorder.

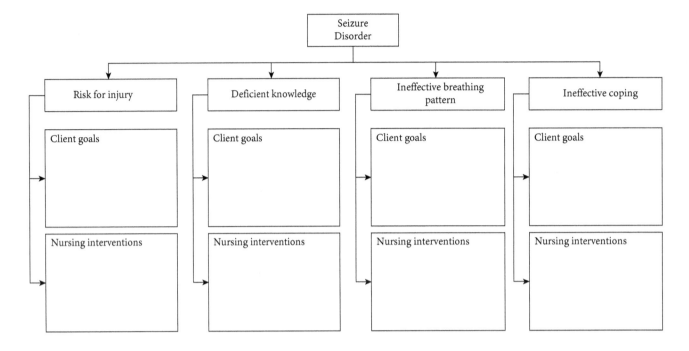

Define Status Epilepticus:

_____

_____

_____

_____

What Is an Aura?

_____

_____

_____

_____

Section I. Application Exercise 7

During the p.m. shift, the client's mother runs to the nursing station. She states, "I think she is having a seizure!" The nurse runs into the client's room and finds the client exhibiting tonic-clonic movements, loss of consciousness, and excessive salivation. After 2 minutes, the tonic-clonic movements cease. From the interventions below, determine a priority nursing diagnosis and prioritize what the nurse should do for the client and mother.

Priority Nursing Diagnosis _____

Nursing Interventions

Assess for any injury   _____

Calm the mother down   _____

Turn client to the side   _____

Assess the client's orientation   _____

Check airway   _____

Notify health care provider   _____

Document occurrence   _____

Nursing Management

Assessment:

_____
_____
_____
_____

Diagnosis:

_____
_____
_____
_____

Interventions:

_____
_____
_____
_____

Section I. Application Exercise 8

The client is being discharged. Implement a teaching plan for the client and mother.

Discharge Teaching	Rationale
Medication Regimen	
Restrictions	

Safety	
Follow-up Care	

Case Scenario: David is a 20-year-old college student who lives in the dorms at his school. He is an athletic scholar and is very popular on campus. He is seen in the campus health center with complaints of stiff neck, headaches, chills, and some nausea and vomiting. History is negative for the meningitis vaccine. He is told to go immediately to the local medical center's emergency department. Upon arrival to the emergency department, blood samples and cerebrospinal fluid sample are taken.

Vital signs: T: 100.1, P: 92, R: 24, BP: 132/86.

Tidbit

Meningitis is more prevalent in communities where people live near one another. It is more prevalent in developing countries.

Meningitis

Define:

_____

_____

_____

_____

Section I. Application Exercise 9

Lab studies reveal that the client has meningitis B caused by *Neisseria meningitidis*. What are the risk factors that indicate the client has been susceptible to this type of meningitis?

_____

_____

_____

Cause/Risk Factors:

_____

_____

_____

_____

Manifestations:

_____

_____

_____

_____

Kernig's Sign:

_____
_____
_____
_____

Brudzinski's Sign:

_____
_____
_____
_____

Section I. Application Exercise 10

The client is immediately started on IV antibiotics. He is not sure how he could've gotten sick. The client states, "I eat right and work out all the time. I should not be sick." As the nurse, developing a teaching plan to address the concerns of the client.

Learning Needs Assessment: "Knowledge deficit" regarding _____ (fill in blank).

Defining Characteristics: r/t (circle one or more)

New Knowledge	**Incomplete Knowledge**	**Incorrect Knowledge**
Cognitive limitation	Lack of recall	Limited exposure to information
Limited practice of skill	Developmental stage	

Goal: Client will verbalize or demonstrate.

_____

Outcome Criteria	Information Provided	Evaluation
Examples: Client will identify, list, define, describe, explain, or demonstrate …	Write actual words the nurse will use to provide information.	Was the initial individual assessment accurate? Were the outcome criteria appropriate to the learning goal? Was the teaching method appropriate? Which outcomes were achieved? Which were not achieved, if any?
Client will _____ _____ _____ _____ _____		

Medication Management:

_____
_____
_____
_____

Nursing Management

Assessment:

_____
_____
_____
_____

Diagnosis:

_____
_____
_____
_____

Interventions:

_____
_____
_____
_____

Encephalitis

Tidbit

Anyone can be affected by encephalitis, irrespective of age, sex, or ethnicity. Every year, 500,000 children and adults are affected by encephalitis; that is one person every minute.

Section I. Application Exercise 11

Using the word list, complete the encephalitis concept map below.

West Nile	Fever
EEG	Bloodwork
Antiviral	CSF Sample
CT Scan	Acyclovir
Lyme Disease	Muscle Spasms
ICP	Anti-inflammatory
Antiviral	Paresthesia
Change in Level of Consciousness	Ganciclovir
Herpes Simplex	Anticonvulsant
Coma	Headache

Autoimmune Response   MRI
Corticosteroid   Nuchal Rigidity
Inflammation of the Brain   Death
Photophobia

Encephalitis Concept Map

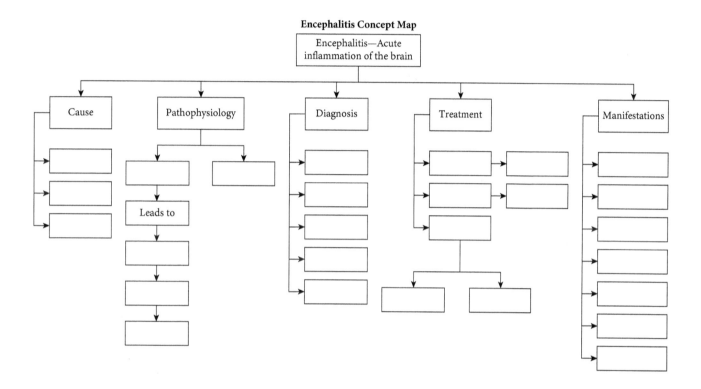

Nursing Management

Assessment:

_____

_____

_____

_____

Diagnosis:

_____

_____

_____

_____

Interventions:

_____

_____

_____

_____

Case Scenario: A 79-year-old female presents to the health care provider's office with abnormal movement in her upper and lower extremities. She states this has been getting worse over the last year. She states that she notices involuntary moments when she is sitting and has experienced the inability to balance herself when walking. The client is alert and oriented. Medical history reveals a healthy individual with no underlying conditions

Vital signs: T: 98, P: 86, R: 24, BP: 136/88.

Parkinson's Disease

Tidbit

About 1 million Americans are thought to have Parkinson's disease. This is more than those affected by multiple sclerosis (MS), muscular dystrophy (MD), and amyotrophic lateral sclerosis (ALS) combined.

Define:

_____

_____

_____

_____

Pathophysiology:

_____

_____

_____

_____

Section I. Application Exercise 12

Fill in the blanks:

Destruction of _____ leads to _____ amount of dopamine in the brain. This causes an imbalance of excitatory _____ and inhibiting _____ in the corpus striatum. This results in loss of _____ and control of _____ _____.

Manifestations:

Define:

Bradykinesia:

_____

_____

_____

Akinesia:

_____

_____

_____

Postural Instability:

_____

_____

_____

Diagnosis:

_____

_____

_____

_____

_____

_____

Section I. Application Exercise 13

The physical exam and history are normal. The presenting diagnoses confirm the diagnosis of Parkinson's. The client is prescribed levodopa/carbidopa. For each Parkinson's medication, discuss the mechanism of action.

Medication	Mechanism of Action
Dopamine Precursors *Levodopa, levodopa/carbidopa (Sinemet)*	
Dopamine Receptor Agonist *Bromocriptine (Parlodel), cabergoline, pramipexole (Mirapex), ropinirole (Requip, Requip XL), rotigotine (Neuro-transdermal patch)*	

Dopamine Agonist
    Amantadine
    Apomorphine (Apokyn)	

Anticholinergics
    Trihexyphenidyl
    Benztropine (Cogentin)	

Antihistamine *Diphenhydramine*	

Monoamine Oxidase Inhibitors
    Selegline (Eldepryl)
    Rasagline (Azilect)	

Catechol-O-Methyltransferase (COMT) Inhibitors
    Entacapone (Comtan)
    Tolcapone (Tasmar)	

Surgical Management:

_____
_____
_____
_____

Nursing Management:

_____
_____
_____
_____

Section I. Application Exercise 14

Using the following diagnoses, develop a plan of care for the client.

Impaired physical mobility, risk for falls, risk for constipation, risk for dysphagia, powerlessness.

Nursing Diagnosis	Intervention	Rationale
Impaired physical mobility		
Risk for falls		
Risk for constipation		

Risk for dysphagia		
Powerlessness		

Case Scenario: Sara, an 82-year-old female, is seen at the health care provider's office today. She is accompanied by her daughter. The daughter states that she takes care of the client and has noticed that Sara is usually oriented during the day but becomes confused in the evening and is up a lot at night. The daughter also states that the client states she sees things in the night and screams out. History of the client reveals diabetes, hypertension, and COPD. The health care provider does a neurological and physical exam. A CT scan is also ordered.

Delirium and Dementia

Section I. Application Exercise 15

Distinguish each characteristic as being Delirium or Dementia.

Delirium: _____ _____ _____ _____ _____ _____ _____ _____ _____ _____

Dementia: _____ _____ _____ _____ _____ _____ _____ _____ _____ _____

1. Alzheimer's disease is its most common form

2. Acute onset, usually occurs at night

3. Can last months to years

4. Judgment is impaired; difficulty with words

5. Awareness is decreased

6. Is aware of surroundings

7. Memory loss is distant

8. Alertness is normal

9. Orientation may fluctuate

10. May seem lethargic

> **Tidbit**
>
> Delirium is a treatable condition and may coexist with dementia. However, it is sometimes difficult to recognize in people with dementia because it has similar symptoms such as confusion and difficulties with thinking and concentration.

11. Recent memory impairment

12. May exhibit illusions or hallucinations

13. Lasts for hours

14. Progression is abrupt

15. Lasts for months to years

16. Gradual onset

17. May have impaired orientation

18. Psychomotor skills are normal

19. Sleep/wake cycles are reversed

Diagnostic Tests:

_____

_____

_____

_____

Nursing Management:

_____

_____

_____

_____

Section I. Application Exercise 16

The diagnostic exam reveals that the client has delirium. The following nursing diagnoses apply to the client: Impaired memory, risk for injury, wandering, self-care deficit.

Using the nursing diagnoses, develop a plan of care with the client and family for the management of delirium.

Nursing Diagnosis	Intervention	Rationale
Impaired Memory		
Risk for Injury		
Wandering		
Self-care Deficit		

Case Scenario: Mr. Mitchell, a 69-year-old male, was seen by the health care provider. He was brought in by his son, who voiced concerns about the increasing forgetfulness and difficulty with language that has been occurring in the client. The son states, "We have noticed that Dad has trouble remembering names and leaving things where he cannot find them." He states his father has always loved reading the morning financial report since he is a retired businessman, but lately he cannot focus and becomes frustrated. History reveals hypertension and recent smoking cessation after 30+ years.

Vital signs: T: 98.6, P: 86, R: 22, BP: 158/86, pulse oximetry: 98%.

Cognitive tests, along with bloodwork and an MRI, are done to rule out metabolic disease, CVA, stroke, or another cardiac disease or vitamin deficiency.

Alzheimer's Disease

Define:

_____
_____
_____
_____

> *Tidbit*
>
> More than 5 million people are living with Alzheimer's disease. It is the 6th leading cause of death in the United States

Pathophysiology:

_____
_____
_____
_____

Medications:

_____
_____
_____
_____

Section I. Application Exercise 17

There are various medications used for the treatment of Alzheimer's disease. Match the medication with the mechanism of action.

Medication	Mechanism of Action
Cholinesterase inhibitors *Donepezil (Aricept)* *Rivastigmine (Exelon)* *Galantamine (Razadyne)*	Precise mechanism of action is not known, but it is suggested that it binds reversibly with and inactivates acetylcholinesterase butyrylcholinesterase, preventing the hydrolysis of acetylcholine, leading to an increased concentration of acetylcholine at cholinergic synapses. Blockade of current flow through channels of N-methyl-d-aspartate (NMDA) receptors—a glutamate receptor subfamily broadly involved in brain function reducing excitotoxicity.
N-methyl-D-aspartate receptor antagonist *Memantine (Namenda)*	Binds reversibly to acetylcholinesterase, inhibits the hydrolysis of acetylcholine, thus increasing the availability of acetylcholine at the synapses, enhancing cholinergic transmission.

Nursing Management:

_____
_____
_____
_____

Section I. Application Exercise 18

Alzheimer's is a devastating disease to the client and family. The nurse does teaching with the client and family. Give the rationale for each of the nursing actions.

Nursing Actions	Rationale
Use a calm, positive voice when speaking to the client.	
Use diversional activities during the day.	
Assist with toileting and bathing.	
Implement safety measures.	
Assist with meals.	

Use clock and calendar.	
Encourage support groups for family.	
Monitoring system for home.	
Secure dangerous materials in home.	

Section II. Peripheral Nervous System Disorders

Case Scenario: A 65-year-old male presents at the health care provider's office with complaints of double vision and drooping eye. He states this has been going on for about a year now, but he thought it was just stress. He also states he has had some difficulty with speech, chewing and swallowing at times, and upper arm weakness that has gotten worse within the last few months. The health care provider refers him to the neurologist.

The neurologist performs a neurological exam and does a blood workup on the client.

Vital signs: T: 98.8, P: 88, R: 26, BP: 146/78, pulse oximetry: 98%.

Myasthenia Gravis (MG)

Define:

_____

_____

_____

_____

_____

_____

Pathophysiology:

_____

_____

_____

_____

_____

_____

> *Tidbit*
>
> The name myasthenia gravis, which is Latin and Greek in origin, means "grave, or serious, muscle weakness."

Section II. Application Exercise 1

Cranial nerves play a role in the diagnosis of MG. Match the cranial nerve with its purpose.

Purpose	Cranial nerve
Controls head, neck, and shoulder movement	IX (glossopharyngeal)
	X (vagus)
Plays a role in function Controls the tongue (movement, tastes, temperature) Blood pressure	XI (spinal accessory)
Innervates head, neck, abdominal, and thoracic organs	XII (hypoglossal)
Controls gag reflex, swallowing	

Manifestations:

_____
_____
_____
_____
_____
_____

Diagnostic Tests:

_____
_____
_____
_____
_____
_____

Section II. Application Exercise 2

The neurologist's exams show muscle weakness, and bloodwork is positive for antibodies associated with MG. Define the various tests used to diagnose MG.

Electromyography (EMG)

_____
_____
_____
_____

Tensilon Test

_____
_____
_____
_____

Serological Test

_____
_____
_____
_____

CT Scan

_____
_____
_____
_____

Medical Management:

_____
_____
_____
_____

Section II. Application Exercise 3

A diagnosis is made of MG for the client. The client is prescribed a cholinesterase inhibitor medication, Mestinon 60 mg q 4 hours, and prednisone 15 mg q d. The client asks what these medications are for. Develop a drug card with purpose and nursing considerations for the client.

Medication	Purpose	Nursing Considerations
Anticholinesterase Inhibitor *Pyridostigmine (Mestinon)*		
Corticosteroid *Prednisone, Deltasone, Prednicot*		

Plasmapheresis:

_____
_____
_____
_____

IV Immunoglobulin G:

_____
_____
_____
_____

Surgical Management:

_____
_____
_____
_____

Complications

Myasthenia Crisis:

_____
_____
_____
_____

Cholinergic Crisis:

_____
_____
_____
_____

Dietary Recommendations:

_____
_____
_____
_____

Nursing Management:

_____
_____
_____
_____

Section II. Application Exercise 4

The following nursing diagnoses apply to the client:

- Ineffective airway clearance
- Impaired verbal communication
- Risk for aspiration
- Activity intolerance

Choose two priority nursing diagnoses and develop a nursing plan of treatment.

Nursing Diagnosis	Client Goals	Nursing Intervention	Rationale
1.			
2.			

Case Scenario: Jesse, a 25-year-old male, presents to the emergency department with progressive weakness x 5 days. He states currently he is unable walk. The client states that he had an episode of food poisoning 2 weeks ago and was told he had gastroenteritis due to *Campylobacter jejuni*. The client has no significant health history. A neurological workup, MRI, EMG, serum electrolytes, CBC, and lumbar puncture are done.

Vital signs: T: 98.0, P: 86, R: 20, BP: 140/86, pulse oximetry: 98%.

Tidbit

According to the CDC, many studies have been done to see if flu vaccines may cause GBS. In most studies, no link was found between the flu vaccine and GBS. However, two studies did suggest that about 1 more person out of 1 million people vaccinated with seasonal flu vaccine may develop GBS.

Guillain-Barré Syndrome (GBS)

Define:

_____

_____

_____

_____

Pathophysiology:

_____

_____

_____

_____

Manifestations:

What is the pattern of weakness that is seen in clients?

_____

_____

_____

_____

Medical Management:

_____

_____

_____

_____

Section II. Application Exercise 5

Diagnostic tests reveal Guillain-Barré. The treatment plan for the client includes intravenous immunoglobulin and plasmapheresis. Discuss the mechanism of action for these two methods of treatment.

Intravenous Immunoglobulin (IVIG)

Mechanism of Action:

_____

_____

_____

_____

Plasmapheresis

Mechanism of Action:

_____
_____
_____
_____

Dietary Management:

_____
_____
_____
_____

Nursing Management:

_____
_____
_____
_____

Section II. Application Exercise 6

The client is admitted to the neurological unit. The nurse has orders given by the health care provider to carry out. Prioritize the orders for the nurse to implement.

Orient client to room	_____
Document assessment	_____
Administer immunoglobulin	_____
Assess IV site	_____
Perform respiratory assessment	_____
Assess for pain	_____
Do neuro checks q 2 hours	_____
Perform ROM q shift	_____
Turn and reposition patient q 2 hours	_____

Assessment:

_____
_____
_____

Diagnosis:

_____
_____
_____

Interventions:

_____
_____
_____

Evaluation:

_____
_____
_____

Case Scenario: A 52-year-old woman is seen in her health care provider's office with complaints of facial pain for several months. She states the pain began after she had a root canal. She states the pain is worse when she eats or drinks and has difficulty smiling. The client has a history of hypertension. Labs ordered: CBC, sedimentation rate, and MRI. Neurological assessment done.

Vital signs: T: 98.6, P: 86, R: 22, BP: 136/74.

Trigeminal Neuralgia (TN)

Define:

_____
_____
_____

Pathophysiology:

Classic (TN1):

_____
_____
_____

Atypical (TN2):

_____
_____
_____

Manifestations:

_____
_____
_____

Diagnostic Studies:

_____
_____
_____

Medical Management:

_____
_____
_____

Section II. Application Exercise 7

Diagnostic and lab tests rule out any lesions, tumors, or vascular problems. The client is diagnosed with trigeminal neuralgia. The health care provider orders the antiseizure medication Tegretol. Develop a drug card for the medication listing the purpose, mechanism of action, and nursing considerations.

Tegretol
Purpose
Mechanism of Action
Side Effects
Nursing Considerations

Other Medications:

Baclofen

Amitriptyline or Nortriptyline:

_____
_____
_____

Surgical Management

Percutaneous Rhizotomy:

_____
_____
_____

Stereotactic Radiosurgery:

_____
_____
_____

Microvascular Decompression:

_____
_____
_____

Nursing Management:

_____
_____
_____

Section II. Application Exercise 8
Create a concept map for care of the client with trigeminal neuralgia.

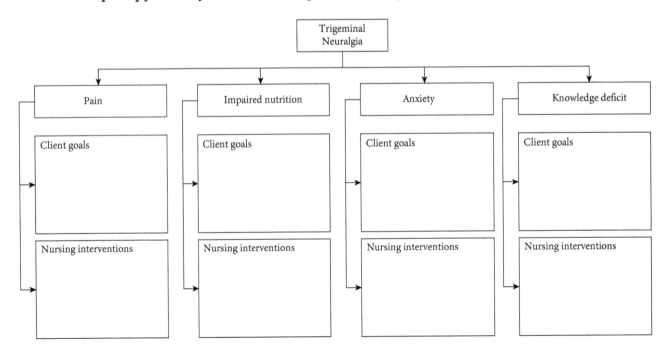

Case Scenario: Jake, a 35-year-old male, is seen by the neurologist. He has been very anxious and is having progressively involuntary movements to his arms and legs over the past year. He also states that chewing and swallowing have become difficult lately. He has had to take a leave of absence from his job due to these symptoms. The client reveals that his family has a history of Huntington's disease, but he was never tested for it. He is worried that he may have the disease. He states, "I am engaged to be married, and I have never told my fiancée about this disease."

Huntington's Disease

Define:

_____

_____

_____

_____

> *Tidbit*
>
> Oscar Waters first described the disease in 1841 and in 1872, George Huntington conducted further research about the disease—hence the name Huntington's disease.

Section II. Application Exercise 9

Why is Jake so worried about his symptoms?

_____

_____

_____

Pathophysiology:

_____

_____

_____

_____

_____

_____

Manifestations:

_____

_____

_____

_____

Section II. Application Exercise 10

Jake decides to have genetic testing. He tests positive for Huntington's disease. What does this mean for Jake?

_____
_____
_____

Diagnosis:

_____
_____
_____

Medical Treatment:

_____
_____
_____

Section II. Application Exercise 11

There is no cure for this disease. The health care provider prescribes several medications that may help the client manage the disease. Complete the chart below on the medications for Huntington's.

Monoamine Depletory	Purpose	Mechanism of Action
Tetrabenazine (Xenazine)		
Antipsychotics		
Haloperidol (Haldol)		
Risperidone (Risperdal)		
Benzodiazepines		
Diazepam (Valium)		
Clonazepam (Klonopin)		
Aripripazole (Abilify)		

Nursing Management:

_____
_____
_____
_____

Section II. Application Exercise 12

The goal of nursing management is to help the client manage and provide reassurance in managing the disease. Using the following diagnosis, create a plan of care for the client. Include a collaborative approach in your care of the client.

- Anxiety
- Knowledge deficit
- Risk for falls
- Imbalanced nutrition
- Ineffective health management

Nursing Diagnosis	Intervention	Rationale

Section III. Spinal Cord Disorders

Case Scenario: A 40-year-old woman was admitted to the emergency department after a fall from a ladder at her home. She is stating that she cannot move her legs and is very anxious. A thorough neurological exam was done in the ambulance on the way to the hospital. Respiratory function is intact. The spine was immobilized. An X-ray, CT scan, or MRI was done.

Vital signs: T: 99.0, R: 24, P: 70, BP: 100/58.

Spinal Cord Injury

Define:

_____
_____
_____
_____

Pathophysiology

Primary Injury:

_____
_____
_____
_____

Secondary Injury:

_____
_____
_____
_____

Classification

Complete Injury:

_____
_____
_____

Incomplete Injury:

_____
_____
_____
_____

Manifestations:

_____
_____
_____

Section III. Application Exercise 1

Manifestations are related to the level of injury. The client's tests reveal a spinal cord injury at the T5 level. Complete the table for each injury level and write the functional loss.

Spinal Cord Injury Level	Functional Loss
C1–C4	
C4, C5	
C5, C6	
C6, C7	
C7, C8	
T1, T5	
T6, T12	

Diagnosis:

Medical Management:

Nonoperative Interventions:

Surgical Therapy:

Medication Management:

Vasopressors

Purpose:

Dopaminergics

Purpose:

_____
_____

Sympathomimetics

Purpose:

_____
_____

Complications

Spinal Shock:

_____
_____
_____
_____

Neurogenic Shock:

_____
_____
_____
_____

Autonomic Dysreflexia:

_____
_____
_____
_____

Halo/Brace Problems:

_____
_____
_____
_____

Section III. Application Exercise 2

The body experiences various complications as a result of a spinal injury.

Discuss how each body system is affected.

Integumentary Complications:

_____
_____
_____

Respiratory Complications:

_____
_____
_____

Gastrointestinal Complications:

_____
_____
_____

Cardiovascular Complications:

_____
_____
_____

Musculoskeletal Complications:

_____
_____
_____

Genitourinary Complications:

_____
_____
_____

Nursing Management:

_____
_____
_____

Section III. Application Exercise 3

The client was taken to surgery for stabilization of the spinal cord. A spinal fusion was done for repair of the injured vertebrae. The surgery was uneventful, and the client is in the PACU.

Vital signs: T: 97.6, P: 76, R: 16, BP: 98/60.

IV fluids of 0.9 NS running at 125ml/hr. Foley catheter in place. Surgical site is covered with dry dressing. Client is stable and is sent to the unit. Prioritize the nursing care that the nurse can delegate to the unlicensed assistive personnel (UAP) and what the nurse should do for the following orders:

	UAP	Nurse
Encourage use of incentive spirometer	_____	_____
Perform passive ROM q shift	_____	_____
Assess surgical site	_____	_____
Monitor for pain	_____	_____
Neuro checks q 2 hrs.	_____	_____
Assess breath sounds	_____	_____
Reposition and maintain alignment	_____	_____
Assess IV site	_____	_____
Monitor SCD compression device	_____	_____
Assist with clear liquid diet	_____	_____
Assess bowel sounds	_____	_____
Monitor I&O	_____	_____

Case Scenario: Harry, a 58-year-old chef, has been experiencing chronic pain in his lower back. On his annual physical at the health care provider's office, he verbalizes pain and muscle spasms to his lower back. He states he stands a lot during the day at his job. He states that his stamina and the ability to move from a sitting to standing position is becoming difficult, especially in the morning. He states he has been taking naproxen sodium 400 mg twice a day with some relief. History reveals 30+ years of smoking and hypertension.

Vital signs: T: 98.8, P: 82, R: 22, BP: 142/86, pulse oximetry: 98%, Ht: 6'4", Wt: 286 lbs.

Diagnostic test ordered: CT scan, EMG.

Low Back Pain

Etiology/Pathophysiology:

_____

_____

_____

_____

_____

_____

_____

Tidbit

According to the American Chiropractic Association, worldwide, back pain is the single leading cause of disability, preventing many people from engaging in work as well as other everyday activities. One-half of all working Americans admit to having back pain symptoms each year.

_____
_____
_____

Manifestations:

_____
_____
_____
_____

Diagnostic Tests

CT Scan:

_____
_____
_____
_____

Electromyography:

_____
_____
_____
_____

Diskogram:

_____
_____
_____
_____

Magnetic Resonance Imaging:

_____
_____
_____
_____

Nerve Conduction Study:

_____
_____
_____
_____

Myelogram:

_____

_____

_____

_____

X-rays:

_____

_____

_____

_____

Medical Management:

_____

_____

_____

_____

Section III. Application Exercise 4

The client has the CT scan and EMG done, which show some loss of spine curvature and reduced range of motion. The health care provider implements a combination of medication management and alternative practices including physical therapy. NSAIDs are the first line of choice. The client has been taking naproxen with little relief. Discuss below the other medications used to treat low back pain.

Medication	Mechanism of Action

Muscle Relaxants
   Carisoprodol (Soma), Cyclobenzaprine (Flexeril),
   Methocarbamol (Robaxin), Metaxalone (Skelexin),
   Diazepam (Valium)	

Corticosteroids Prednisone, cortisone, hydrocortisone	

Anticonvulsants
   Gabapentin (Neurontin), Pregabalin (Lyrica),
   topiramate (Topamax), Carbamazepine (Tegretol)	

Opioids Morphine, codeine, oxycodone	

Tricyclic Antidepressants
   Amitriptyline (Elavil), Nortriptyline (Pamelor),
   Imipramine (Tofranil)	

NSAIDs
   Aspirin, Ibuprofen, ketorolac tromethamine
   (Toradol), naproxen	

Local Anesthetics Lidocaine	

Surgical Management

Nerve Blocks:

_____
_____
_____
_____

TENS:

_____
_____
_____
_____

Laminectomy:

_____
_____
_____
_____

Diskectomy:

_____
_____
_____
_____

Spinal Fusion:

_____
_____
_____
_____

Nursing Management:

_____
_____
_____
_____

Section III. Application Exercise 5

The health care provider gives the following orders:

- Flexeril 5 mg po tid
- Naproxen 200 mg bid prn
- Physical therapy referral
- Teach client on managing low back pain
- Increase fluid intake
- Weight management

Develop a teaching plan the nurse will give to the client.

Teaching Plan	Rationale
Medication Administration	
Nonpharmacological Pain Relief Measures	
Weight Management	
Fluids	

Case Scenario: A 52-year-old male is seen by the health care provider with pain to his neck and radiating to his arm. He states he has had this pain for several months, but the pain has gotten worse over the last few weeks. He takes Advil for pain twice a day with little relief. No significant history noted.

Vital signs: T: 97.8, P: 84, R: 20, BP: 136/70, pulse oximetry: 98%.

Neurological exam done along with MRI and X-ray.

Herniated Nucleus Pulposus

Etiology/Pathophysiology:

_____
_____
_____
_____
_____
_____
_____
_____
_____
_____

Manifestations:

_____
_____
_____
_____

Diagnostic Tests:

_____
_____
_____
_____

Medical Management:

_____
_____
_____
_____
_____
_____
_____
_____

Surgical Management:

_____
_____
_____

> *Tidbit*
>
> Herniated Nucleus Pulposus is also called bulging disk, compressed disk, herniated intervertebral disk, herniated nucleus pulposus, prolapsed disk, ruptured disk, or slipped disk.

Section III: Application Exercise 6

The client's MRI and X-rays show cervical disk protrusion at C5–C6. The health care provider recommends laminectomy. The client is admitted to the hospital, and the procedure is performed without any complications. The client has an uneventful recovery and is on the unit. Prioritize the care the nurse will give to the client.

- _____ Place pillows under legs while supine
- _____ Assess vital signs, especially respiratory status
- _____ Assist with turning and repositioning
- _____ Administer oxycodone 5 mg q 4 hr prn
- _____ Assess pain
- _____ Encourage coughing and deep breathing
- _____ Inspect surgical site
- _____ Monitor neurological status
- _____ Monitor bowel and bladder status

Nursing Management:

_____

_____

_____

_____

Section III. Application Exercise 7

Use the following nursing diagnoses to develop a plan of care for the client being discharged.

- Self-Care Deficit
- Impaired Home Maintenance
- Pain
- Impaired Mobility

Nursing Diagnosis	Intervention	Rationale
Impaired mobility		
Pain		

Self-care deficit		
Impaired home maintenance		

Case Scenario: A 27-year-old female was seen in the outpatient clinic with complaints of some loss of vision and pain in her eyes. She states she has had some double vision for about 24 hours now. She also verbalized some weakness in her arms. She was given a neurological exam and an MRI. History reveals no other health problems.

Vital signs: T: 98.6, P: 78, R: 18, BP: 118/78, pulse oximetry: 100%.

Diagnostic tests: Blood tests to rule out inflammatory or autoimmune disease, vitamin deficiency, and an MRI.

Multiple Sclerosis (MS)

Define:

_____

_____

_____

_____

Etiology/Pathophysiology:

_____

_____

_____

_____

Section III. Application Exercise 8

The bloodwork was negative for any inflammatory or autoimmune disease. The MRI shows a lesion on the brainstem. No treatment was given at that time. Two months later, the client returns to the outpatient center with increased weakness and fatigue. Her gait is also unsteady. A second MRI was done, which revealed another lesion in the right cerebral part of the brain. She is diagnosed with relapsing-remitting multiple sclerosis. Discuss the differences in the types of MS.

Types

Relapsing-Remitting:

_____
_____
_____
_____

Secondary Progressive:

_____
_____
_____
_____

Progressive Relapsing:

_____
_____
_____
_____

Primary Progressive:

_____
_____
_____
_____

Manifestations:

_____
_____
_____
_____

Diagnostic Tests:

_____
_____
_____

Medical Management:

_____

_____

_____

_____

Medication Management:

_____

_____

_____

_____

Section III. Application Exercise 9

Since there is no cure for MS, the disease is managed through medication. The client will be managed on Interferon, corticosteroids, muscle relaxants, and laxatives. For each class of medication, list the mechanism of action.

Class	Mechanism of Action

Immunomodulators
   Interferon beta 1a (Avonex, Rebif)
   Interferon beta 2a (Betaseron, Extavia)	

Immunomodulator—synthetic protein
   Glatiramer (Copaxone)
   Fingolimod (Gilenya)	

Immunosuppressants
   Natalizumab (Tysabri)
   Mitoxantrone (Novantrone)	

Muscle relaxants and antispasmodics
   Baclofen (lioresal, Kemstrol)
   Tizanidine (Zanaflex)	

Corticosteroids *Prednisone, cortisone, hydrocortisone, methylprednisone sodium succinate (Solu-Medrol)*	
Stool softeners *Docusate (Colace)*	
Anticholinergics, antispasmodics *Oxybutynin chloride (Ditropan)*	

Analeptics
   Modafinil(Provigil)
   Armodafinil (Nuvigil)	

Antimuscarinics *Tolterodine (Detrol)*	

Osmotic laxatives *Milk of magnesia, Miralax, Lactulose*	
Stimulant laxatives *Dulcolax, Senokot, Correctol*	
Anticonvulsants *Phenytoin (Dilantin), Gabapentin (Neurontin),* *Pregabalin (Lyrica), Topiramate (Topamax),* *Carbamazepine (Tegretol)*	

Nursing Management:

_____
_____
_____
_____

Create a concept map for care of the client with multiple sclerosis.

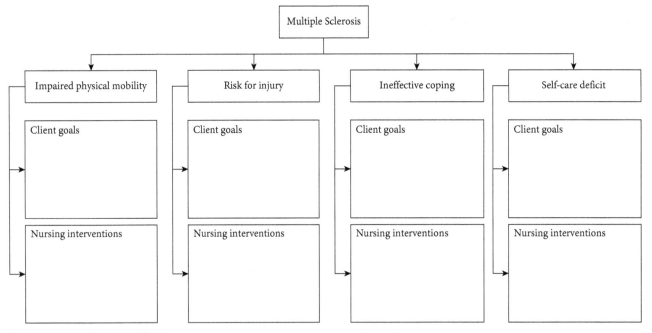

Amyotrophic Lateral Sclerosis (ALS)

Section III. Application Exercise 10

Use the word list to complete the concept map for ALS.

Word List **for ALS Concept Map**

Impaired verbal communication	Risk for aspiration
Ineffective breathing pattern	Ineffective coping
Upper/lower motor neurons degenerate	Cell death

CT scan	Paralysis
Gradual degeneration of motor neurons	Blood studies
Anticholinergics	Occupational therapy
Stiffness	Slurred speech
Analeptics	Medications
Brain loses ability to initiate movement	Spasticity
Flaccidity	MRI
Muscle weakness, atrophy	Speech therapy
Physical therapy	Lumbar puncture
Laxatives	Benzothiazole
Nutritional support	Dysphagia
Gradual muscle weakness and atrophy	Muscle relaxants
Antidepressants	History/physical
Risk for injury	Ineffective airway clearance

Using the word list, complete the concept map for ALS.

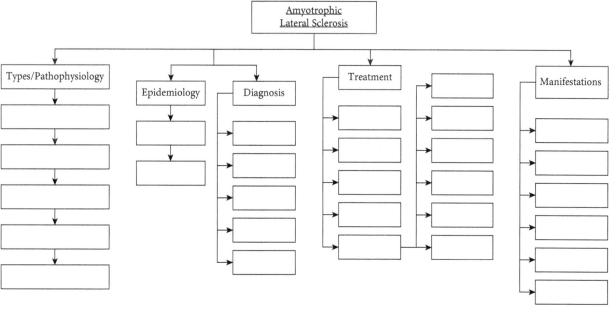

Write the interventions for each nursing diagnosis.

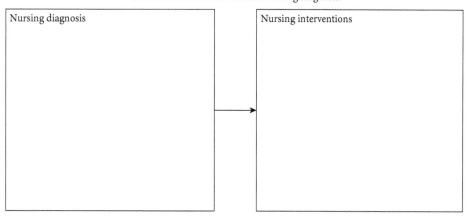

Critical Thinking Questions

1. When assessing the body functions of a patient with increased ICP, what should the nurse assess first?

   a. Corneal reflex testing

   b. Pupillary reaction to light

   c. Extremity strength testing

   d. Circulatory and respiratory status

2. A patient is admitted to the hospital with possible bacterial meningitis. During the initial assessment, the nurse questions the patient about a recent history of what?

   a. Mosquito or tick bites

   b. Chickenpox or measles

   c. Cold sores or fever blisters

   d. An upper respiratory infection

3. The nurse is preparing to admit a newly diagnosed patient experiencing tonic-clonic seizures. What could the nurse delegate to unlicensed assistive personnel (UAP)?

   a. Complete the admission assessment.

   b. Assess the details of the seizure event.

   c. Obtain the suction equipment from the supply cabinet.

   d. Place a padded tongue blade on the wall above the patient's bed.

4. The nurse explains to a patient newly diagnosed with MS that the diagnosis is made primarily by

   a. Spinal X-ray findings

   b. T-cell analysis of the blood

   c. Analysis of cerebrospinal fluid

   d. History and clinical manifestations

Chapter 15

Perioperative

Introduction

This chapter will discuss perioperative nursing and its incumbent responsibilities.

PERIOPERATIVE NURSING ENCOMPASSES the total operative experience. Working closely with surgeons, anesthesiologists, and surgical technicians, the nurse functions in various roles in the surgical process and is responsible for the functioning of the entire surgical suite and the client's experiences throughout the surgical process. From completing the preoperative assessment to the postoperative discharge, the nurse is responsible for the safety and well-being of the client. This chapter will focus on each phase of the surgical process and the responsibilities of the nurse throughout each phase in caring for the client.

Learning Objectives of This Chapter

Upon completion of this chapter, the student should be able to:

- Describe problems of the preoperative, intraoperative, and postoperative phases.
- Examine the nursing role and responsibility in the physical, psychological, and educational preparation of the surgical patient.
- Identify common preoperative and postoperative medications.
- Interpret significant data related to the surgical patient.
- Describe client safety outcomes and measures in the preoperative, intraoperative, and postoperative phases.

Self Study Guide
Complete the following as you listen to the lecture and/or refer to your textbook.

Section I. Preoperative Nursing

Perioperative Nursing

Define:

_____

Preoperative Phase: _____

Intraoperative Phase: _____

Postoperative Phase: _____

Classification of Surgical Procedures

Type	Description and Examples
Admission status Ambulatory (outpatient) Same-day admit Inpatient	
Seriousness Major Minor	
Urgency Elective Urgent Emergent	
Purpose Reconstructive Diagnostic (Exploratory) Palliative Cosmetic	
Ablative	
Minimally Invasive	
Telesurgery (Robotic)	

Surgical Terminology

Term	Interpretation with Example
Anastomosis	
-ectomy	
Lysis	
-orrhaphy	
-oscopy	
-ostomy	
-otomy	
-pexy	
-plasty	

Case Scenario: Curtis is a 26-year-old male who is being seen by the health care provider for a preoperative workup. He is scheduled to have a tonsillectomy. He has a history of smoking and strep throat, with his most recent episode 2 weeks ago. He has allergies to latex and penicillin. States that he has pain in his throat that is currently 6/10.

Vital signs: T: 98.8, P: 78, R: 22, BP: 128/76, pulse oximetry: 98%.

Preoperative Checklist

Purpose:

_____
_____
_____

Components of the Checklist:

_____
_____
_____
_____
_____
_____
_____
_____
_____
_____

Section I. Application Exercise 1

The nurse must complete an assessment and preop checklist. One of the things included is the consent for surgery. Complete the chart for the components of the informed consent.

Components of Informed Consent
Procedure:
Anesthesia:
Blood Products:

What must be done if the client cannot sign the consent form?

_____

_____

_____

List the responsibilities of the nurse and physician regarding informed consent.

Physician:

_____

_____

_____

Nurse:

_____

_____

_____

Advance Directives

Living Will:

_____

_____

_____

Do Not Intubate:

_____

_____

_____

Do Not Resuscitate:

_____

_____

_____

Section I. Application Exercise 2

The nurse is preparing the client for surgery. The client is asked his name and the nurse verifies it using the identification band. His date of birth is incorrect. The nurse immediately calls the admissions office to send up a corrected ID band. The "time-out" procedure is done to make sure that the correct information is identified. Fill in the blanks regarding the "time-out" procedure.

During the preop phase, the client's _____ is looked at and compared to a verbalization of the client's name. The client should also state the _____ that is to be performed.

This process is repeated during the _____ phase immediately prior to the first incision.

Health Assessment

Subjective Data

Psychosocial Assessment:

_____
_____
_____
_____
_____
_____
_____
_____

Past Health History:

_____
_____
_____
_____
_____
_____
_____
_____
_____
_____
_____
_____

Medications:

_____
_____
_____
_____
_____
_____
_____
_____
_____
_____

Surgical and Anesthesia History:

_____
_____
_____

_____
_____
_____
_____

Allergies:

_____
_____
_____
_____
_____
_____
_____

Miscellaneous Drug/Alcohol Use:

_____
_____
_____
_____
_____
_____
_____

Review of Systems

Cardiovascular:

_____
_____
_____
_____
_____

Respiratory:

_____
_____
_____
_____
_____

Neurological System:

_____
_____

_____
_____
_____

Genitourinary:

_____
_____
_____
_____
_____

Hepatic:

_____
_____
_____
_____

Integumentary:

_____
_____
_____
_____
_____

Musculoskeletal:

_____
_____
_____
_____
_____

Gastrointestinal:

_____
_____
_____
_____
_____

Immune System:

_____
_____

_____
_____
_____

Gerontological Considerations:

_____
_____
_____
_____
_____

Section I. Application Exercise 3

The client has his preop checklist done and the client is ready to be transferred to the OR suite. Prioritize the interventions that must be done by the nurse prior to transfer.

_____ Document last oral intake

_____ Remove and secure jewelry

_____ Establish time-out

_____ Insert IV line

_____ Teach deep breathing

_____ Obtain set of vitals

_____ Prep skin and bowel

_____ Teach client what to expect

Section II. Intraoperative Nursing

Department Layout

Unrestrictive:

_____
_____
_____
_____

Semi-restrictive:

_____

_____

_____

Restrictive:

_____

_____

_____

_____

Holding Area:

_____

_____

_____

_____

Operating Room:

_____

_____

_____

_____

Section II. Application Exercise 1

Surgical team roles: State the role and circle whether it is sterile or nonsterile.

Scrub Nurse (Sterile, Nonsterile):

_____

_____

_____

_____

LPN/Surgical Technologist (Sterile, Nonsterile):

_____

_____

_____

_____

Circulating Nurse (Sterile, Nonsterile):

_____
_____
_____
_____

Surgeon and Assistant (Sterile, Nonsterile):

_____
_____
_____
_____

Registered Nurse First Assistant (Sterile, Nonsterile):

_____
_____
_____
_____

Anesthesia Care Provider (Sterile, Nonsterile):

_____
_____
_____
_____

Anesthesiologist:

_____
_____
_____
_____

Nurse Anesthetist:

_____
_____
_____
_____

Section II. Application Exercise 2

Match the surgical attire with the purpose.

Worn to protect feet from injury; usually covered	Goggles
Prevents the shedding of hair, squamous cells, and/or dandruff onto the scrub suit	Surgical gowns
Protects the patient and the hands against infection	Masks
Made of material to protect against blood and fluids	Footwear
Protects the mucous membranes of the eyes, nose, and mouth during procedures in which the possibility of splashes or sprays of blood, body fluids, and other secretions could occur	Gloves
	Caps

Section III. Anesthesia

Anesthesia

Define:

_____
_____
_____
_____
_____

Types of Anesthesia

   1. General:

_____
_____
_____

Inhalation of Gases:

_____
_____
_____

IV Agents:

_____
_____
_____

Tidbit

The first public demonstration of modern anesthesia was on October 16, 1846 ("Ether Day"). William T. G. Morton and surgeon John Collins Warren made anesthesia history at Massachusetts General Hospital with the successful use of diethyl ether "anesthesia" to prevent pain during surgery.

Muscle Relaxants:

_____
_____
_____

Complications of General Anesthesia:

- _____

   _____

- _____

   _____

- _____

   _____

- _____

   _____

- _____

   _____

- _____

   _____

- _____

   _____

Malignant Hyperthermia:

_____
_____
_____

Section III. Application Exercise 1

Use the word list to complete the concept map for malignant hyperthermia.

Hypercarbia dantrolene	Increased intracellular calcium ion concentration
Myoglobinuria	Muscle relaxant
Hypermetabolic state caused by exposure to a triggering agent	Dark urine
Hypermetabolism	Glycolysis
Volatile gases, succinylcholine	Remove blankets
Cold body lavage	IV infusion of cold normal saline
Rigidity of skeletal muscles	Cool client
Hyperthermia (late)	Hypercarbia
Hypoxemia	Acidosis
Sustained muscle contractions	Hyperthermia
Unexplained tachycardia	Tachycardia

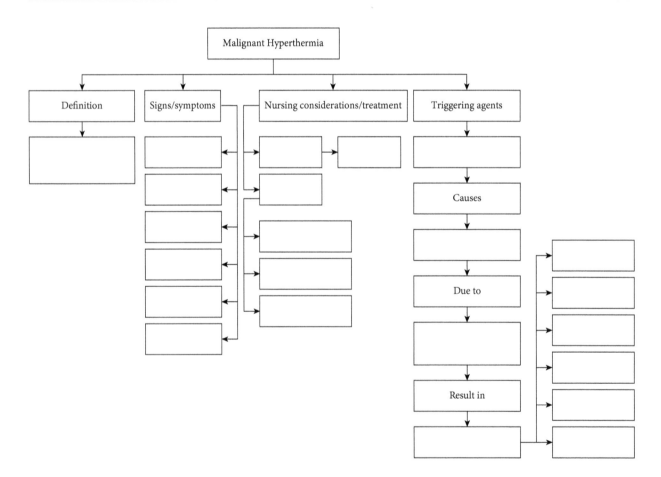

2. Regional:

_____
_____
_____

Spinal:

_____
_____
_____
_____

Epidural:

_____
_____
_____
_____

Caudal:

_____
_____
_____
_____

Nerve Blocks:

_____
_____
_____
_____

Complications of Spinal Anesthesia:

_____
_____
_____
_____

3. Local:

_____
_____
_____

Amides:

_____

_____

_____

_____

Esters:

_____

_____

_____

_____

4. Monitored:

_____

_____

_____

_____

_____

Airway Management

Define:

_____

_____

_____

_____

Section III. Application Exercise 2

Match the type of airway device with its purpose.

Purpose	Type of Airway
Protects the airway and the client can breathe spontaneously; best method to manage airway	Face mask
Helps maintain spontaneous breathing, covers mouth mask	Laryngeal airway
Used for brief surgeries and not as irritating to the airway	Endotracheal tube

Section IV. Positioning the Client

Purpose of Positioning:

_____

_____

_____

Section IV. Application Exercise 1

State the indication for each surgical position.

Supine: _____

Prone: _____

Jackknife: _____

Low Lithotomy: _____

Trendelenburg: _____

Reverse Trendelenburg: _____

Fowler's: _____

High Lithotomy: _____

Lateral: _____

Positioning Devices:

_____

_____

_____

_____

Positioning Complications

Pressure Injury:

_____

_____

Situations That May Cause Pressure Injury:

_____
_____
_____
_____

Client at Risk for Complications Due to Positioning:

_____
_____
_____
_____

Section IV. Application Exercise 2

Using the following diagnoses, create a plan of care for the surgical client.

- Risk for infection related to _____
- Knowledge deficit related to _____
- Risk for injury related to _____
- Risk for aspiration related to _____
- Risk for impaired circulation related to _____
- Risk for impaired skin integrity related to _____

Nursing Diagnosis	Intervention	Rationale

Section V. Postoperative

Case Scenario: Mrs. Olson, a 56-year-old female, had a total abdominal hysterectomy and is admitted into the post-anesthesia care unit for monitoring. She is drowsy but is responsive to her name. IV of D5LR infusing at 125 ml/hr. O_2 at 2l via nasal cannula. Foley catheter draining clear yellow urine.

Vitals: T: 98.8, P: 86, R: 22, BP: 142/84, pulse oximetry: 97%. Rates pain as a 6 out of 10.

Lungs sound clear bilaterally. Small 4x4 dressing noted to lower abdominal area. Sequential compression devices on legs. The client was medicated for pain with morphine and fentanyl prior to admission to the PACU.

Postoperative Care

Post-anesthesia Care Unit (PACU)

Purpose:

_____

_____

_____

_____

PACU Progression

Phase I:

_____

_____

_____

_____

Phase II:

_____

_____

_____

_____

Phase III:

_____

_____

_____

_____

Nursing Management:

_____

_____

_____

_____

Section V. Application Exercise 1

The nurse is responsible for managing the client when they are admitted to the PACU. Provide rationale for each area of assessment.

Respiratory:

_____

_____

_____

Vital Signs:

_____

_____

_____

Neurological:

_____

_____

_____

Pain:

_____

_____

_____

Fluid Status:

_____

_____

_____

Dressing/Incision:

_____

_____

_____

Diagnostic Tests in the PACU

Purpose:

_____

_____

_____

_____

_____

Section V. Application Exercise 2

Match the implication with each diagnostic test.

Glucose	Done to evaluate clotting abnormalities
BUN/Creatinine	Low values indicate blood loss
White blood cell count	May be decreased due to fluid/blood loss and dehydration
PT/PTT	Decrease may be responsible for decreased level of consciousness
Serum sodium and potassium	Increase may indicate infection
Hemoglobin/hematocrit	May be abnormal due to overhydration, blood loss, or fluid loss

Methods of Pain Management

Wong-Baker FACES:

_____

_____

_____

NSAIDs:

_____
_____
_____

Acetaminophen:

_____
_____
_____

Opioids:

_____
_____
_____

Local Anesthetics:

_____
_____
_____

Alternative Therapies:

_____
_____
_____

Section V. Application Exercise 3

The client was also admitted with a patient-controlled analgesia (PCA) pump. She is to receive 0.2 mg of hydromorphone with a lockout of 10 minutes. She is still a bit drowsy but can follow and understand commands. She is complaining of discomfort and doesn't know how to use the pump.

Discuss and teach the client about the use of the pump and indicate the nursing responsibilities while monitoring the patient using the PCA.

Purpose	

How the Pump Works	

Nursing Responsibilities
 	
  Pain
 	
  Sensation
 	
  Respiratory
 	
    Rate
 	
    Pulse Oximetry
 	
    Lung Sounds	

Postoperative Complications

Nausea/Vomiting:

_____
_____
_____
_____

Respiratory:

_____
_____
_____
_____

Cardiovascular:

_____
_____
_____
_____

Neurological:

_____
_____
_____
_____

Gastrointestinal:

_____
_____
_____
_____

Genitourinary:

_____
_____
_____
_____

Alterations in Temperature:

_____
_____
_____
_____

Integumentary:

_____
_____
_____

Dehiscence:

_____

Evisceration:

_____

Discharge from PACU Criteria:

_____
_____
_____

_____

_____

Section V. Application Exercise 4

The client is stable and is ready to be transferred to the unit from the PACU. The PACU nurse must give a clear and concise report to the unit nurse. List the information that the PACU nurse must give.

- _____
- _____
- _____
- _____
- _____
- _____
- _____
- _____

Section V. Application Exercise 5

The following orders are given to the unit nurse for the postop client: continue IV fluids of D5LR at 100 ml/hr. Vitals q 4 hours; discontinue PCA pump and give Percocet 1–2 tabs q 4–6 hours prn pain; assess dressing and reinforce as needed with sterile 4x4 but do not change monitor for pain; discontinue Foley catheter; monitor output; up in chair this evening. Soft diet and advance as tolerated.

Client is alert and oriented and states her pain is a 4 out of 10. Prioritize the care the nurse will give.

Intervention		Rationale for Prioritization
Assess dressing	_____	_____
Assess for vitals and pain	_____	_____
Orient client to room	_____	_____
Get up in chair	_____	_____
Discontinue Foley	_____	_____
Administer pain meds	_____	_____
Order food tray	_____	_____
Discontinue PCA pump	_____	_____
Assess IV site and change IV fluids	_____	_____
Do head-to-toe assessment	_____	_____

Gerontological Considerations

Respiratory:

_____

_____

_____

Cardiac:

_____
_____
_____

Gastrointestinal:

_____
_____
_____

Genitourinary:

_____
_____
_____

Integumentary:

_____
_____
_____

Musculoskeletal:

_____
_____
_____

Nutrition:

_____
_____
_____

Psychosocial:

_____
_____
_____

Critical Thinking Review Questions

1. Which statement, if made by a new circulating nurse, is inappropriate?

    a. I will assist in preparing the operating room for the patient.

    b. I will remain gloved while performing activities in the unsterile field.

    c. I will assist with suturing of incisions and maintaining hemostasis as needed.

    d. I will count the number of sponges, needles, instruments, and other supplies during the procedure.

2. A patient scheduled to undergo an abdominal hysterectomy surgery under general anesthesia asks the nurse, "Will I be asleep for the whole procedure?" Which response by the nurse is most appropriate?

    a. You will be given medication through your IV line first. I will check with the anesthesia care provider.

    b. I am not sure what method of anesthesia will be used. Should I ask your surgeon?

    c. General anesthesia is now given in many ways, so you may or may not need a mask over your face.

    d. A tube will be inserted into your throat to deliver a gas that will put you to sleep.

3. When caring for a preoperative patient on the day of the surgery, which actions included in the plan of care can the nurse delegate to unlicensed assistive personnel (UAP)? (*Select all that apply.*)

    a. Teach incentive spirometer use.

    b. Explain preoperative routine care.

    c. Obtain and document baseline vital signs.

    d. Remove nail polish and apply pulse oximeter.

    e. Transport the patient by stretcher to the operating room.

4. In the post-anesthesia care unit (PACU), a patient's vital signs are blood pressure 120/72, pulse 76, respirations 16, and SpO_2 94%. The patient is drowsy but awakens easily. Which action should the nurse take first?

    a. Place the patient in a side-lying position.

    b. Encourage the patient to use incentive spirometer.

    c. Prepare to transfer the patient to a clinical unit.

    d. Increase the rate of the postoperative IV fluids.

Chapter 16

Pharmacology in Nursing

Introduction

This chapter will focus on some basic pharmacological concepts you will need to assist you in understanding and applying your knowledge in medication administration.

A s a nursing student, you were required to take many prerequisite courses to enter your nursing program. These courses likely included chemistry, biology, microbiology, and pathophysiology. One reason for these science courses is to help you understand pharmacology, as many of these basic sciences are necessary for medication administration.

As a caregiver and as a nurse, it will be your responsibility to assess the patient before administering medications and after administration. In order to do this, you must be able to have a solid and detailed understanding of the responsibilities of drug administration. You must be able to determine what the medication is for and why the patient has been prescribed the medication. Learning the therapeutic and pharmacological classifications, trade and generic names as well as being able to identify prescription and nonprescription medications is vital. Being able to recognize restrictions regarding controlled substances and how they are to be given is another important aspect and responsibility of the nurse. It is your responsibility to prevent and minimize any harm associated with administering medications by carrying out these fundamental principles of medication administration. Pharmacology teaches about how drugs are given, why they are given, how they travel throughout the body, how the body responds to them, and how they exit the body.

Learning Objectives of This Chapter

Upon completion of this chapter, the student should be able to:

- Define pharmacological terms
- Identify the meaning of complementary and alternative medications
- Differentiate between over-the-counter medications and prescription medications
- Define terms related to medication administration
- Identify how medications are excreted

- Describe the rights of medication administration and label checks
- Differentiate the types of therapeutic responses to medications
- Identify terms related to drug reactions
- Discuss the terms controlled substance and teratogens

Section I

Match the term with the definition

Term	Definition
Pharmacology	1. A chemical agent capable of producing biologic responses within the body.
Therapeutics	2. A substance that has the potential to cause a defect in an unborn child during the mother's pregnancy.
Duration of drug action	3. Chemically synthesized drugs that are closely related to biologic medications having already received U.S. Food and Drug Administration (FDA) approval.
Pharmacotherapy	4. Refers to the way a drug works at the molecular, tissue, or body system level.
Peak plasma level	5. Role of heredity in drug response.
Medication	6. Concerned with the prevention of disease and treatment of suffering.
Pharmacokinetics	7. Helpful in predicting a substance's physical and chemical properties.
Anaphylaxis	8. After a drug is administered, it is called anaphylaxis.
Adverse	9. Short and easy to remember and is assigned by the company marketing the drug.
Therapeutic classification	10. The study of medicine.
Mechanism of action	11. Undesirable effect.
Chemical name	12. The application of drugs for the purpose of treating diseases and alleviating human suffering.
Biosimilar drugs or biosimilars	13. Contains more than one active generic ingredient.
Generic name	14. One of the primary alerts for identifying extreme adverse drug reactions discovered during and after the review process.
Adherence	15. A physiologic or psychologic need for a substance.
Combination drug	16. Agents naturally produced in animal cells, by microorganisms, or by the body itself.
Pharmacologic classification	17. Method of organizing drugs is based on their therapeutic usefulness in treating particular diseases or disorders.
Black box warnings	18. Less complicated and easier to remember than chemical names.
Dependence	19. Physical signs of discomfort.
Adverse effect	20. Refers to how a medicine changes the body.

Term	Definition
Potency	21. Nontherapeutic reaction to a drug.
Maintenance doses	22. A severe type of allergic reaction that involves the massive, systemic release of histamine and other chemical mediators of inflammation that can lead to life-threatening shock.
Therapeutic	23. The study of drug movement throughout the body.
Side effect	24. Occurs when the medication has reached its highest concentration in the bloodstream.
Biologics	25. Taking a medication in the manner prescribed by the health care provider or, in the case of OTC drugs, following the instructions on the label.
Onset of drug action	26. Amount of time a drug maintains its therapeutic effect.
Drug	27. A higher amount of drug often given only once or twice to "prime" the bloodstream with a sufficient level of drug.
Idiosyncratic responses	28. Given to keep the plasma drug concentration in the therapeutic range.
Loading dose	29. Represents the amount of time it takes to produce a therapeutic effect after drug administration.
Allergic reaction	30. An unfavorable drug reaction.
Pharmacodynamics	31. The magnitude of maximal response that can be produced from a particular drug.
Efficacy	32. Unpredictable and unexplained drug reactions.
Trade name	33. Will produce a therapeutic effect at a lower dose, compared with another drug in the same class.
Withdrawal	34. Acquired hyper-response of body defenses to a foreign substance (allergen).
Pharmacogenetics	35. How a drug produces its physiologic effect in the body.
Teratogen	36. Desirable effects.

Section II

Describe the difference between over the counter and prescription medications.

_____

_____

_____

_____

_____

Why would one be preferred over the other?

_____

_____

_____

_____

_____

Complementary and Alternative Medicines (CAM)

Define: _____

_____

_____

List some CAM therapies

1. _____

2. _____

3. _____

4. _____

5. _____

6. _____

7. _____

8. _____

9. _____

Drug-to-Drug Interactions

Define and differentiate between the following terms related to medication administration:

A. Synergism _____

_____

B. Antagonism _____

_____

C. Addition _____

_____

D. Displacement _____

_____

Medication Metabolism and Excretion

What is the significance of the liver and kidneys for medications?

- Kidney _____

_____

_____

_____

- Liver _____
_____
_____
_____

What if the client has a kidney injury or liver cirrhosis?

_____
_____
_____
_____

Section III

Medication Administration

Match the five rights with their definitions

Must give to the right person.	Right medication
Provide the correct drug for the condition.	Right dose
Use the correct route of administration to provide the drug.	Right time
Use the appropriate dose.	Right patient
Understand when to administer a drug and when not to.	Right route

Name three additional rights.
1. _____
2. _____
3. _____

What are the three label checks?
1. _____
2. _____
3. _____

Why are the three label checks important?

_____
_____
_____

Section IV

Therapeutic Responses to Medications

Define the following:

Onset of the medication

_____
_____
_____

Peak plasma level

_____
_____
_____

Duration of the medication

_____
_____
_____

What is meant by a loading dose of a medication? Intermittent? What is the purpose of administering a drug in this manner?

_____
_____
_____
_____
_____
_____

Section V

Drug Reactions

There are possible scenarios the nurse must be aware of regarding administration of certain medications. These medications may have a high potential for addiction. It is important to know and recognize these terms.

Match the description with its definition

Dependence	The patient has an intense desire to continue to use the drug.
Physical dependence	A need for a drug, either physical or physiological.
Withdrawal	Occurs with the repeated use of a drug; patient's physical condition adapts to the drug.
Psychological dependence	When drug is no longer available, the patient experiences discomfort.

Describe the unfavorable drug reactions in each scenario as either a **side effect, allergic reaction,** or **anaphylaxis.**

1. Samuel Jones, age 16, has been prescribed a medication to treat his bacterial infection. After the first dose, Samuel develops a runny nose and a rash on his neck and arms. This is a (an)

    _____

2. Maria Lopez, age 32, has been prescribed a medication to treat her GERD. Maria has noticed that when she takes the medication, she feels anxious and has difficulty breathing. This is a (an)

    _____

3. Brady Collins, age 56, has a diagnosis of hypertension. He has been prescribed a beta blocker. When visiting his heath care provider, he verbalizes that he has some swelling in his lower extremities. This is a (an)

    _____

Controlled Substances

These are substances that have the potential to be abused by the patient prescribed the medication. They are categorized as scheduled drugs. These schedules are numbered I to V.

Describe what these schedules mean and what is the highest number of the scheduled drugs that have the potential for being abused.

_____
_____
_____
_____
_____
_____

Teratogens

These are substances that can cause a defect to the fetus during pregnancy. They are categorized as A, B, C, D, and X.

Describe what these categories mean and what is the highest number of the categorized drugs that have the potential for being abused.

_____
_____
_____
_____
_____
_____

Critical Thinking Questions

1. A nurse has the following responsibilities when administering medications. (*Select all that apply.*)

    a. Make sure the five rights are implemented with each med pass.

    b. Verify that the health care provider's orders are accurate.

    c. Monitor the patient for any possible reactions.

    d. Obtain baseline vitals prior to medication administration.

    e. Answer any questions that the patient may have about the medication.

2. The nurse is preparing to administer medication to Mrs. Connor. As the medications are reviewed, she tells the nurse that she is allergic to a certain medication on the list. The nurse should: (*Select all that apply.*)

    a. Notify the health care provider and the pharmacy of the allergy.

    b. Tell her, "It's ok, the doctor would not have prescribed the medication if she thought there was an allergy."

    c. Document the allergy on the patient's chart.

    d. Place an allergy bracelet on the patient.

    e. Give the medication anyway.

3. When should a "STAT" order be given to a patient?

    a. After the nurse makes sure the patient can tolerate the drug.

    b. Within 5 min after the order is received.

    c. Within 30 min after receiving the order.

    d. Before the shift ends.

4. A patient is scheduled for an outpatient procedure in the am. The health care provider gives an order to have the patient NPO after midnight prior to the procedure. The patient has a history of diabetes and takes an oral antidiabetic medication daily. What is the best action for the nurse to implement in relation to administration of the oral antidiabetic medication?

    a. Follow all of the health care provider's orders.

    b. Clarify with the physician if the medication can be given.

    c. Tell the patient to go ahead and just take the medication because it is important due to her diabetes.

    d. Tell the patient to only take half of the dose.

5. A patient has a history of chronic kidney failure and is on dialysis 3 days a week. What must the nurse monitor for with the patient?

   a. The therapeutic effect of the medication.

   b. Allergies of the patient.

   c. A synergistic effect of medications.

   d. Assess for increased risk for drug toxicity.

6. What must the nurse do if the wrong medication has been administered? (*Select all that apply.*)

   a. Fill out an incidence report and put it in the chart.

   b. Assess the patient for any adverse reactions.

   c. Report the error to the nurse manager.

   d. Document the error in the chart.

   e. Notify the hospital's risk management department.

7. You are the nurse for a difficult patient. She drills every nurse about what medications she is receiving each time she is scheduled to take her medicines. As you give the medications to her, she asks to see them. She states, "I have never seen this orange pill before." What should the nurse do?

   a. Reassure her that the pill is not new, and she should take it.

   b. Verify the Medication Administration Record (MAR) and make sure this is a prescribed medication.

   c. Let her know that sometimes different brands may change the colors of medications.

   d. Let the patient call her health care provider.

8. A patient is prescribed azithromycin. There is a loading dose to be given to be followed by a maintenance dose for 7 days. The patient asks why there is a loading dose and what does it mean. The nurse best response would be

   a. A loading decreases the number of doses that you will take.

   b. A loading dose decreases the risk of an adverse reaction.

   c. A loading dose results in lower dosages needed to reach desired effects.

   d. A loading dose is a higher amount of drug, often given only once or twice to prepare the bloodstream with a sufficient level of drug so that therapeutic levels are reached sooner.

Appendix

Chapter 1 Answer Key

Answers to Critical Thinking Questions

1. **B.** IV KCl is administered at a maximal rate of 10 mEq/hr. Rapid IV infusion of KCl can cause cardiac arrest. Although the preferred concentration for KCl is no more than 40 mEq/L, concentrations up to 80 mEq/L may be used for some patients. KCl can cause inflammation of peripheral veins, but it can be administered by this route. Cardiac monitoring should be continued while patient is receiving potassium because of the risk for dysrhythmias.

2. **A.** Hypertonic solutions cause water retention, so the patient should be monitored for symptoms of fluid excess. Crackles in the lungs may indicate the onset of pulmonary edema and are a serious manifestation of fluid excess. Bounding peripheral pulses, peripheral edema, or changes in urine output are also important to monitor when administering hypertonic solutions, but they do not indicate acute respiratory or cardiac decompensation.

3. **A.** The pH and HCO_3 indicate that the patient has a metabolic acidosis. The ABGs are inconsistent with the other responses.

4. **C.** Hypomagnesemia is associated with alcoholism. Protein intake would not have a significant effect on magnesium level. OTC laxatives (such as milk of magnesia) and use of multivitamin/mineral supplements would tend to increase magnesium levels.

5. **C.** Respiratory alkalosis, partially compensated.

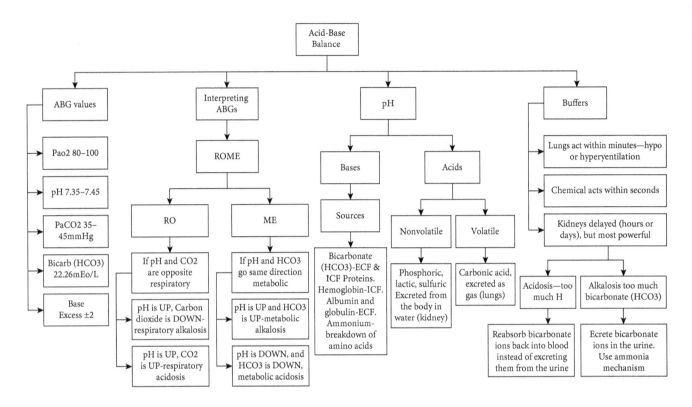

Acid-Base Concept Map

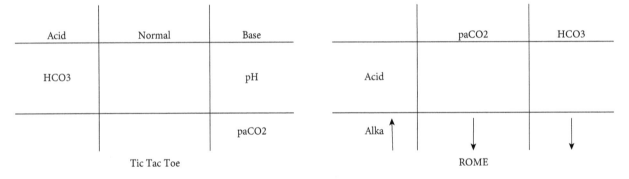

Chapter 2 Answer Key

Section IV. Key to Critical Thinking Questions

1. **A, C, D, E.** Offering small, frequent, high-calorie, high-protein feedings, encouraging generous fluid intake, turning, and teaching effective coughing techniques will assist in thinning secretions and clearing the airway.

2. **C.** Getting the client to verbalize his or her feeling is effective for determining how to assist them in ways to have more interactions with others.

3. **B, C, E, G.** Resting, eating small meals, high-fiber foods, and foods with carbohydrates are the best nutritive intervention for patients with COPD.

4. **B, C, D.** When assessing the activity of the COPD client, asking about sleep cycles, activities of daily living, and other activities is important for the nurse to recognize to develop a plan of care for the client.

Section III. Application Exercise 2

Key to Critical Thinking Questions

1. **B.** Decreased lung sounds and decreased lung expansion could indicate the development of a complication such as empyema or pus in the pleural space. The nurse should check the client's oxygen saturation and notify the provider. Infection can also move into the bloodstream and result in sepsis, so quick treatment is needed.

2. **B.** Increasing fluids has been proven to decrease the thickness of secretions, thus allowing them to be expectorated quickly. The other interventions would not be as effective.

3. **C.** The client who works in a day care facility and is infected with *Streptococcus pneumoniae* may have a drug-resistant pneumonia. It is extremely important that this organism does not spread to other clients; the client should be isolated.

4. **B.** Although age is a factor in the development of community-acquired pneumonia, other lifestyle and exposure factors increase the risk to a greater extent than age. Two conditions that heavily predispose to the development of pneumonia are cigarette smoking and alcoholism. Dietary choices typically do not predispose to the development of pneumonia. Cigarette smoking interferes with the ciliary function of removal of invasive materials. Alcoholism usually results in unbalanced nutrition, as well as decreased immune function. A middle-aged adult, an older adult with wheezing induced by exercise, and a young adult vegetarian would not be at risk for community-acquired pneumonia because they have no predisposing conditions.

Section IV. Application Exercise 4

Key Critical Thinking Questions

1. **B.** Orange-colored body secretions are an expected side effect of rifampin. The other statements are true.

2. **B.** A high-efficiency particulate-absorbing (HEPA) mask, rather than a standard surgical mask, should be used when entering the patient's room because the HEPA mask can filter out 100% of small airborne particles. All of the other interventions are appropriate.

3. **B.** The first action should be to determine whether the patient has been compliant with drug therapy because negative sputum smears would be expected if the TB bacillus is susceptible to the medications and if the medications have been taken correctly. Assessment is the first step in the nursing process. Depending on whether the patient has been compliant or not, different medications or directly observed therapy may be indicated. The other options are interventions based on assumptions until an assessment has been completed.

4. **D.** Teach the patient how to minimize exposure to close contacts and household members. Homes should be well ventilated, especially the areas where the infected person spends a lot of time. While still infectious, the patient should sleep alone, spend as much time as possible outdoors, and minimize time in congregate settings or on public transportation.

Section V. Application Exercise 4

Key to Critical Thinking Questions

1. **B.** Bronchoconstriction and increased mucus productions are most important to address as a priority. The anxiety will decrease as airway is cleared. Patient teaching will be done after treating the client.

2. **C, D, E.** Elevating head of the bed to semi-Fowler's position, staying with the client, and helping them remain calm and providing rest period is needed to facilitate breathing.

3. **D.** Readings in the yellow zone indicate a decrease in peak flow. The patient should use short-acting b2-adrenergic (SABA) medications. Readings in the green zone indicate good asthma control. The patient should exhale quickly and forcefully through the peak flow meter mouthpiece to obtain the readings. Readings in the red zone do not indicate good peak flow, and the patient should take a fast-acting bronchodilator and call the health care provider for further instructions. Singulair is not indicated for acute attacks but rather is used for maintenance therapy.

4. **B.** The goal for treatment of an asthma attack is to keep the oxygen saturation >90%. The other patient data may occur when the patient is too fatigued to continue with the increased work of breathing required in an asthma attack.

Chapter 3 Answer Key

Key to Critical Thinking Questions

1. **D.** Pallor of the skin or nail beds is indicative of anemia, which would be indicated by a low Hgb level. Platelet counts indicate a person's clotting ability. A neutrophil is a type of white blood cell that helps to fight infection.

2. **D.** Adherence to diet and drug therapy is important for the patient with iron deficiency anemia. To replenish iron stores, the patient may need to take iron therapy for 2–3 months to get hemoglobin levels within normal limits.

3. **C.** Organ meats and green leafy vegetable are high in iron.

4. **B.** Lifelong administration of vitamin B-12 is needed for the patient with pernicious anemia. A typical treatment is 1000 mg of cobalamin (B-12) IM for two weeks and then monthly for life.

Answers to NCLEX Style Questions

1. **B.** Atherosclerosis results from a buildup of fats in the openings of the arteries due to a fatty diet.

2. **D.** Because family history, gender, and age are nonmodifiable risk factors, the nurse should focus on the patient's LDL level. Decreases in LDL will help reduce the patient's risk for developing CAD.

3. **B.** Skim milk, oatmeal, banana, orange juice, coffee are the best selections for a low-cholesterol diet.

4. **A.** Canned foods have a high sodium content, and the patient is correct in stating he or she will give those away.

Concept Map—Angina

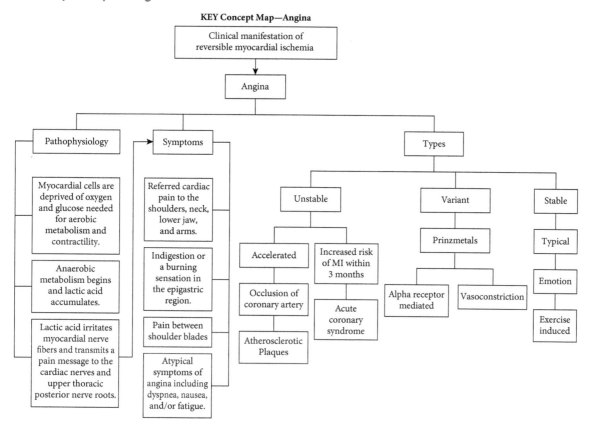

KEY Concept Map—Angina

Medication Management Concept Map

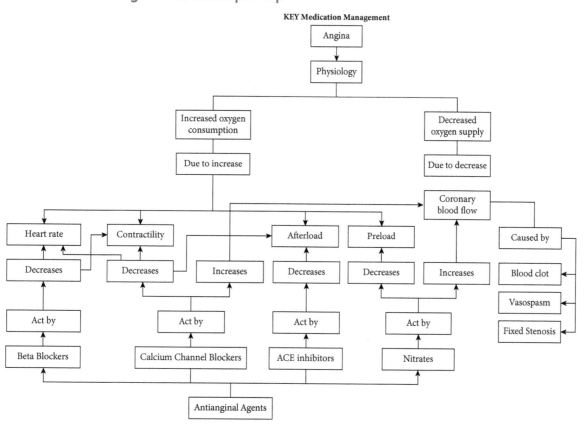

KEY Medication Management

Chapter 4 Answer Key

Key to Critical Thinking Questions

1. **D.** Thrombophlebitis is an inflammatory process that causes a blood clot to form and block one or more veins, usually in your legs. Signs and symptoms include warmth, tenderness, and pain in the affected area; redness and swelling.

2. **D.** Compression of the leg is essential to healing of venous stasis ulcers. High dietary intake of protein, rather than carbohydrates, is needed. Prophylactic antibiotics are not routinely used for venous ulcers. Moist dressings are used to hasten wound healing.

3. **B.** Discoloration of the skin and the absence of hair are indications of arterial insufficiency.

4. **A.** Because the edema associated with venous insufficiency increases when the patient has been standing, shoes will feel tighter at the end of the day. The other patient statements are characteristic of peripheral artery disease.

Chapter 5 Answer Key

Key to Critical Thinking Questions

1. **C.** A transient ischemic attack (TIA) is a stroke that lasts only a few minutes. It happens when the blood supply to part of the brain is briefly blocked. Symptoms of a TIA are a warning sign of a stroke, but do not last as long. They happen suddenly, and include numbness or weakness, especially on one side of the body.

2. **A.** If the stroke occurs in the left side of the brain, the right side of the body will be affected, producing some symptoms such as paralysis or weakness on the right side of the body and aphasia.

3. **C.** A carotid endarterectomy is a procedure in which the artery is opened and obstructing plaque is removed.

4. **A, B, D, E.** It is important to be patient and allow the client to express their needs and allow them to maintain as much independence as possible. Neurological checks should be done more than once a day.

5. **C.** Client assessment indicates rapid breathing and possible hypoxia. To fully assess the respiratory status of the client, it is important to take the pulse oximetry.

6. **A, B, D.** The administration of oxygen improves O_2 saturation and assists in meeting tissue oxygen demands and thereby relieves dyspnea and fatigue.

7. **A.** A commonly prescribed diet for the heart failure client is a 2-gram low-sodium diet. All food high in sodium should be eliminated. Soups are high in sodium content.

8. **A, B, D.** The heart failure patient should implement a regularly scheduled activity and rest regimen to improve outcome and manage the disease.

Chapter 6 Answer Key

Key to Critical Thinking Questions

1. **B.** Tagamet and Zantac are H2 receptor antagonists that decrease gastric acid secretion. Erythromycin and Flagyl are anti-infective medications. Kayexalate is used to treat high blood potassium. Maalox contains aluminum hydroxide and magnesium hydroxide, which act to neutralize or reduce stomach acid for the purpose of relieving the symptoms of indigestion, heartburn, and gastroesophageal reflux disease. Diazide is a combination of a thiazide diuretic (water pill) and a potassium-sparing diuretic is used to treat fluid retention (edema) and high blood pressure (hypertension). Carafate works mainly in the lining of the stomach by sticking to ulcer sites and protecting them from acids, enzymes, and bile salts.

2. **A, B, C, D, E.** All of the interventions would help to stimulate the client's intake.

3. **B.** Clear, cool liquids are usually the first foods started after a patient has been nauseated. Acidic foods such as grape juice, very hot foods, and hot chocolate are poorly tolerated when patients have been nauseated.

4. **C.** GERD is exacerbated by eating late at night, and the nurse should plan to teach the patient to avoid eating at bedtime. The other patient actions are appropriate to control symptoms of GERD.

Chapter 7 Answer Key

Key to Critical Thinking Questions

1. **B.** An initial therapy for an acute exacerbation of inflammatory bowel disease (IBD) is to rest the bowel by making the patient NPO. Metoclopramide increases peristalsis and will worsen symptoms. Cobalamin (vitamin B-12) is absorbed in the ileum, which is not affected by ulcerative colitis. Although a total colectomy is needed for some patients, there is no indication that this patient is a candidate.

2. **A.** Medications are used to bring on remission in patients with inflammatory bowel disease (IBD). Decreased activity level is indicated only if the patient has severe fatigue and weakness. Fluids are needed to prevent dehydration. There is no advantage to enteral feedings.

3. **D.** Abdominal distention is seen in lower intestinal obstruction. Referred back pain is not a common clinical manifestation of intestinal obstruction. Metabolic alkalosis is common in high intestinal obstruction because of the loss of HCl acid from vomiting. Projectile vomiting is associated with higher intestinal obstruction.

4. **D.** One criterion for the diagnosis of irritable bowel syndrome (IBS) is the presence of abdominal discomfort or pain for at least 3 months. Abdominal distention, flatulence, and food intolerance are also associated with IBS, but are not diagnostic criteria.

5. **D.** Avoidance of gluten-containing foods is the only treatment for celiac disease. Corn does not contain gluten, while oatmeal and wheat do.

Chapter 8 Answer Key

Key to Critical Thinking Questions

1. **B.** Tan or gray stools indicate biliary obstruction, which requires rapid intervention to resolve. The other data are not unusual for a patient with this diagnosis, although the nurse would also report the other assessment information to the health care provider.

2. **A.** Asterixis indicates that the patient has hepatic encephalopathy, and hepatic coma may occur. The spider angiomas and right upper quadrant abdominal pain are not unusual for the patient with cirrhosis and do not require a change in treatment. The ascites and weight gain indicate the need for treatment but not as urgently as the changes in neurological status.

3. **B.** Any patient with a history of IV drug use should be tested for hepatitis C. Blood transfusions given after 1992 (when an antibody test for hepatitis C became available) do not pose a risk for hepatitis C. Hepatitis C is not spread by the oral-fecal route and therefore is not caused by contaminated food or by traveling in underdeveloped countries.

4. **A.** Respiratory failure can occur as a complication of acute pancreatitis, and maintenance of adequate respiratory function is the priority goal. The other outcomes would also be appropriate for the patient.

Chapter 9 Answer Key

Answers to Critical Thinking Questions

1. **B.** Acute glomerulonephritis frequently occurs after a streptococcal infection such as strep throat. It is not caused by kidney stones, hypertension, or urinary tract infection (UTI).

2. **C.** Because a 28-year-old patient may be considering having children, the nurse should include information about genetic counseling when teaching the patient. The well-managed patient will not need to choose between hemodialysis and peritoneal dialysis or know about the effects of transplantation for many years. There is no indication that the patient has chronic pain.

3. **B.** The low blood pressure indicates that urosepsis and septic shock may be occurring and should be immediately reported. The other findings are typical of pyelonephritis.

4. **B.** Patients with metabolic acidosis caused by AKI may have Kussmaul respirations as the lungs try to regulate carbon dioxide. Bounding pulses and vasodilation are not associated with metabolic acidosis. Because the patient is likely to have fluid retention, poor skin turgor would not be a finding in AKI.

Chapter 10 Answer Key

Answers to Critical Thinking Questions

1. **C.** To avoid disruption of the suture line, the patient should avoid brushing the teeth for 10 days after surgery. It is not necessary to remain on bed rest after this surgery. Coughing is discouraged because it may cause leakage of cerebrospinal fluid (CSF) from the suture line. The head of the bed should be elevated 30 degrees to reduce pressure on the sella turcica and decrease the risk for headaches.

2. **B.** Acromegaly causes an enlargement of the hands and feet. Head injury and family history are not risk factors for acromegaly. Tremors and anxiety are not clinical manifestations of acromegaly.

3. **C.** When water is retained, the serum sodium level will drop below normal, causing the clinical manifestations reported by the patient. The hematocrit will decrease because of the dilution caused by water retention. Urine will be more concentrated with a higher specific gravity. The serum chloride level will usually decrease along with the sodium level.

4. **C.** Nocturia occurs as a result of the polyuria caused by diabetes insipidus. Edema, excess fluid volume, and fluid retention are not expected.

5. **B.** Oral calcium supplements are used to maintain the serum calcium in normal range and prevent the complications of hypocalcemia. Whole grain foods decrease calcium absorption and will not be recommended. Bisphosphonates will lower serum calcium levels further by preventing calcium from being reabsorbed from bone. Kidney stones are not a complication of hypoparathyroidism and low calcium levels.

Endocrine Concept Map Key

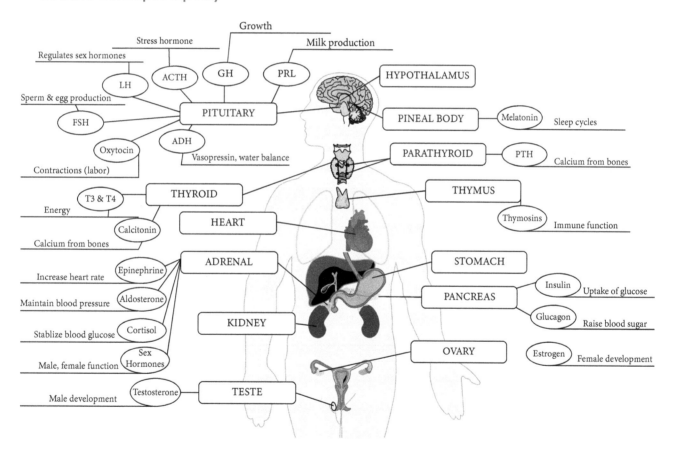

Chapter 11 Answer Key

Key to Critical Thinking Questions

1. **C.** The management of DKA is similar to that of HHS except that HHS requires greater fluid replacement because of the severe hyperosmolar state. Bicarbonate is not usually given in DKA to correct acidosis

unless the pH is less than 7.0 because administration of insulin will reverse the abnormal fat metabolism. Total body potassium deficit is possible in both conditions, requiring monitoring and possible potassium administration, and in both conditions glucose is added to IV fluids when blood glucose levels fall to 250 mg/dl (13 mmol/L).

2. **A, C, E, F.** Manifestations of hyperglycemia include abdominal cramps, polyuria, weakness, fatigue, and headache. The headache may also be seen with hypoglycemia that is manifested by the remaining options.

3. **D.** Complete or partial loss of protective sensation of the feet is common with peripheral neuropathy of diabetes, and patients with diabetes may suffer foot injury and ulceration without ever having pain. Feet must be inspected during daily care for any cuts, blisters, swelling, or reddened areas.

4. **D.** This glucagon-like peptide (GLP-1) receptor agonist stimulates GLP-1 to increase insulin synthesis and release from the pancreas, inhibit glucagon secretion, slow gastric emptying, and must be injected subcutaneously once every 7 days. The other medications are oral agents (OAs). The mechanism of action for glycemic control for the dopamine receptor agonist is unknown. Dipeptidyl peptidase-4 (DDP-4) inhibitors block the action of the DDP-4 enzyme that inactivates incretin so there is increased insulin release, decreased glucagon secretion, and decreased hepatic glucose production. Sodium-glucose co-transporter 2 (SGLT2) inhibitors block the reabsorption of glucose by the kidney and increase urinary glucose excretion.

Key to Section I. Application Exercise 2

Using the word list, complete the concept map on the process of blood glucose level control.

Word List

- Beta cells release
- Insulin
- Alpha cells release
- Glucagon
- Blood glucose levels rise; glucagon levels decrease

- Blood glucose levels decrease; insulin release decreases
- Liver takes up glucose and stores it as glycogen
- Cells take up more glucose
- Liver breaks down glycogen and releases glucose to the blood

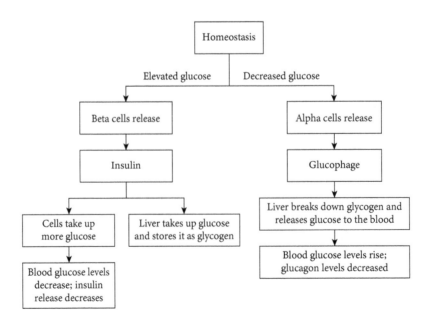

Key to Section IV. Application Exercise 1

Using the word list, complete the concept maps for the dawn phenomenon and the Somogyi effect.

- Results in higher fasting blood glucose levels in a.m.
- Natural release of counterregulatory hormones
- Counterregulatory hormones are released to increase blood glucose
- Liver releases glucose stores to increase blood glucose levels
- Insulin dose given at bedtime
- Body does not have enough insulin to control glucose increase
- Blood glucose levels drop
- Blood glucose level rises

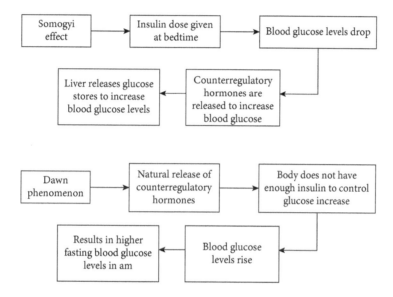

Chapter 12 Answer Key

Answers to Critical Thinking Questions

1. **C.** Comfortable shoes with good support will help decrease the risk for falls. Scatter rugs should be eliminated, not just tacked down. Activities of daily living provide range of motion exercise; these do not need to be taught by a physical therapist. Falls inside the home are responsible for many injuries.

2. **C, D, B, E, A, F.** The initial actions should be to ensure adequate airway, breathing, and circulation. This should be followed by checking the neurovascular condition of the leg (before and after splint application). Application of a splint to immobilize the leg should be done before sending the patient for X-ray examination. The tetanus prophylaxis is the least urgent of the actions.

3. **B.** UAP can be responsible for maintaining the integrity of the traction after it has been established. The RN should assess the extremity and assure manual traction is maintained if the traction device has to be removed and reapplied. Assessment of skin integrity and circulation should be done by the registered nurse (RN).

4. **B.** The patient should be adequately medicated for pain before any attempt to ambulate. Instructions about the benefits of ambulation may increase the patient's willingness to ambulate, but decreasing pain

with ambulation is more important. The presence of an incisional drain or timing of dressing change will not affect ambulation.

Key to Application Exercise 7

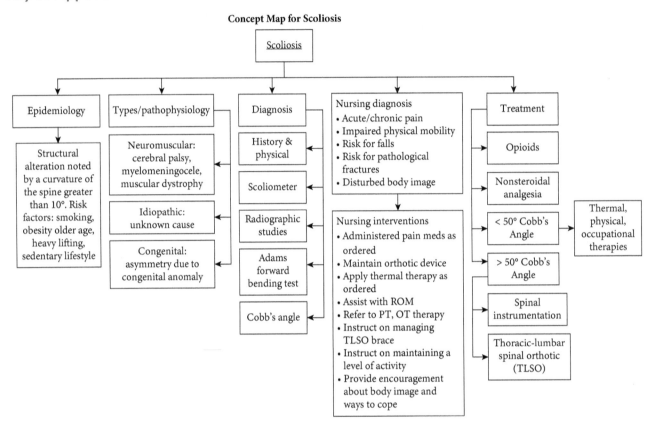

Concept Map for Scoliosis

Chapter 13 Answer Key

Answers to Critical Thinking Questions

1. **D.** All infections of the conjunctiva or cornea are transmittable, and frequent, thorough hand washing is essential to prevent the spread from one eye to another or to other persons. Artificial tears are not normally used for eye infections. Photophobia is not experienced by all patients with eye infections. Warm or cool, not iced, compresses are indicted for some infections.

2. **B.** The patient with dry AMD can benefit from low vision aids despite increasing loss of vision, and it is important to promote a positive outlook by not giving patients the impression that "nothing can be done" for them.

3. **A, C, E, F.** Acute PACG is caused by the lens blocking the papillary opening, which causes loss of central vision with corneal edema. Sudden severe eye pain and nausea and vomiting can occur, and it is initially treated with hyperosmotic oral and IV fluids. Treatment with trabeculoplasty or trabeculectomy or B-adrenergic blockers are associated with POAG.

4. **A, D, E.** Myopia is characterized by excessive light refraction, the image focused in front of the retina, and correction with a concave or divergent lens. Myopic people may have abnormally long eyeballs, not abnormally short ones, which occurs in hyperopia and is corrected with a convex lens. Unequal corneal curvature results in astigmatism.

Key to Section I. Application Exercise 1

There are several diagnostic tests that are done to gather information to determine treatment for ocular disorders. Match the different diagnostic tests with their purpose.

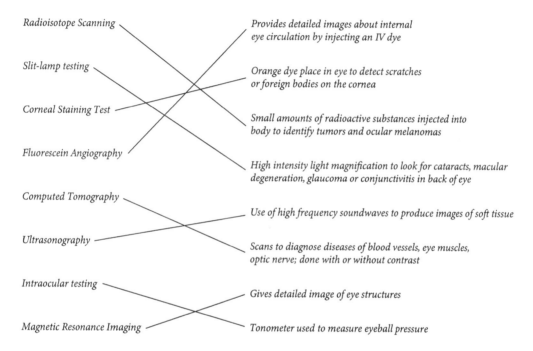

Chapter 14 Answer Key

Answers to Critical Thinking Questions

1. **D.** Of the body functions that should be assessed in an unconscious patient, cardiopulmonary status is the most vital function and gives priorities to the ABCs.

2. **D.** Meningitis is often a result of an upper respiratory infection or a penetrating wound of the skull, where organisms gain entry to the CNS. Epidemic encephalitis is transmitted by ticks and mosquitoes, and non-epidemic encephalitis may occur as a complication of measles, chicken pox, or mumps. Encephalitis caused by the herpes simplex virus carries a high fatality rate.

3. **C.** The UAP is able to obtain equipment from the supply cabinet or department. The RN may need to provide a list of necessary equipment and should set up the equipment and ensure proper functioning. The RN is responsible for the initial history and assess as well as assessing and documenting seizure events. Padded tongue blades are no longer used, and no effort should be made to place anything in the patient's mouth during a seizure.

4. **D.** There is no specific diagnosis for MS. A diagnosis is made primarily by history and clinical manifestations. Certain diagnostic tests may be used to help establish a diagnosis of MS. Positive findings on an MRI include evidence of at least two inflammatory demyelinating lesions in at least two different locations within the central nervous system. Cerebrospinal fluid may have an increased immunoglobulin G and the presence of oligoclonal banding. Evoked potential responses are often delayed in persons with MS.

Key to Section I. Application Exercise 3

Distinguish each characteristic as being delirium or dementia.

Delirium: 2, 3, 5, 9, 10, 12, 13, 14, 19

Dementia: 1, 4, 6, 7, 8, 11, 15, 16, 17, 18, 19

1. Alzheimer's disease is its most common form

2. Acute onset, usually occurs at night

3. Speech is incoherent

4. Judgment is impaired; difficulty with words

5. Awareness is decreased

6. Is aware of surroundings

7. Memory loss is distant

8. Alertness is normal

9. Orientation may fluctuate

10. May seem lethargic

11. Recent memory impairment

12. May exhibit illusions or hallucinations

13. Lasts for hours

14. Progression is abrupt

15. Lasts for months to years

16. Gradual onset

17. May have impaired orientation

18. Psychomotor skills are normal

19. Sleep/wake cycles are reversed

Key to Section I. Application Exercise 12 Concept Map

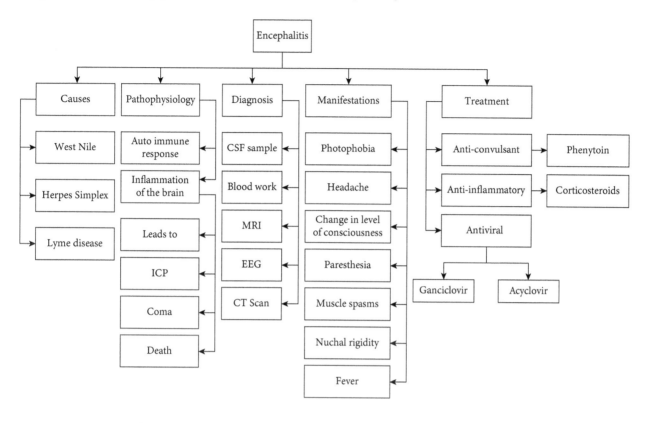

Key to Section I. Application Exercise 13
Fill in the blanks.

Destruction of ***dopaminergic cells in the substantia nigra*** leads to ***decreased*** amounts of dopamine in the brain. This causes an imbalance of excitatory ***acetylcholine*** and inhibiting ***dopamine neurotransmitters*** in the corpus striatum. This results in loss of ***initialing*** and control of ***voluntary movements***.

Key to Section III. Application Exercise 10
Using the word list, complete the concept map for ALS.

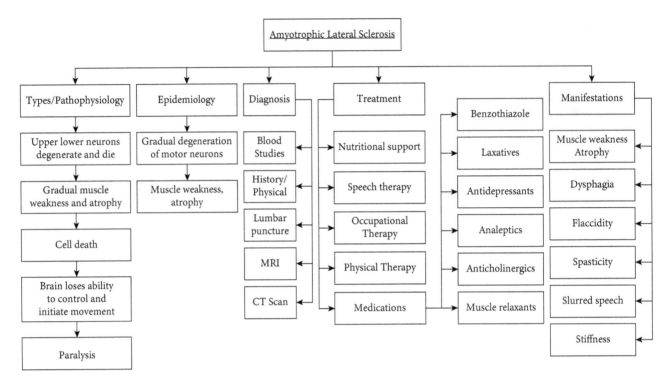

Nursing Diagnoses

- Ineffective airway clearance
- Risk for aspiration
- Ineffective breathing pattern
- Impaired verbal communication
- Risk for injury
- Ineffective coping

Chapter 15 Answer Key

Answers to Critical Thinking Questions

1. **C.** The scrub nurse is responsible for suturing incisions and maintaining homeostasis. All other answer options describe specific types of circulating nurses. The circulating nurse performs activities in the unsterile field and is not scrubbed, gowned, or gloved. The scrub nurse follows the designated scrub procedure, is gowned and gloved in sterile attire, and performs activities in the sterile field.

2. **A.** Routine general anesthesia is usually induced by the IV route with a hypnotic, anxiolytic, or dissociative agent. However, general anesthesia may be induced by IV or by inhalation. The nurse should consult with the anesthesia care provider to determine the method selected for this patient. The anesthesia care provider will select the method of anesthesia, not the surgeon. Inhalation agents may be given through an endotracheal tube or a laryngeal mask airway.

3. **C, D, E.** Obtaining vital signs, removing nail polish, pulse oximeter placement, and transport of the patient are routine skills that are appropriate to delegate. Teaching patients about the preoperative routine and incentive spirometer use requires critical thinking and should be done by the registered nurse.

4. **B.** The patient's borderline SpO$_2$ and drowsiness indicate hypoventilation. The nurse should stimulate the patient and remind the patient to take deep breaths using the incentive spirometer. The lateral position is needed when the patient first arrives in the PACU and is unconscious. Fluid status is stable as evidenced by the stable blood pressure and pulse. The patient is not fully awake and has a low SpO$_2$, indicating that transfer from the PACU to a clinical unit is not appropriate.

Key to Section III. Application Exercise 1

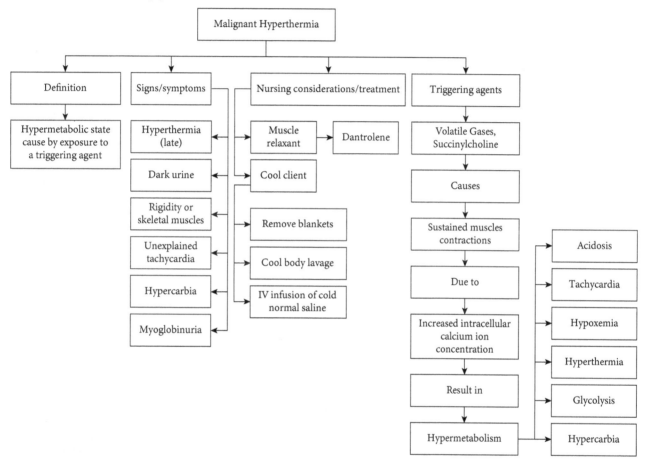

Chapter 16 Answer Key

Key to Section I

	Term	Definition
10.	Pharmacology	1. A chemical agent capable of producing biologic responses within the body.
36.	Therapeutics	2. A substance that has the potential to cause a defect in an unborn child during the mother's pregnancy.
26.	Duration of drug action	3. Chemically synthesized drugs that are closely related to biologic medications having already received U.S. Food and Drug Administration (FDA) approval.

12.	Pharmacotherapy	4. Refers to the way a drug works at the molecular, tissue, or body system level.
24.	Peak plasma level	5. Role of heredity in drug response.
8.	Medication	6. Concerned with the prevention of disease and treatment of suffering.
23.	Pharmacokinetics	7. Helpful in predicting a substance's physical and chemical properties.
22.	Anaphylaxis	8. After a drug is administered, it is called anaphylaxis.
11.	Adverse	9. Short and easy to remember and is assigned by the company marketing the drug.
17.	Therapeutic classification	10. The study of medicine.
35.	Mechanism of action	11. Undesirable effect.
7.	Chemical name	12. The application of drugs for the purpose of treating diseases and alleviating human suffering.
3.	Biosimilar drugs or biosimilars	13. Contains more than one active generic ingredient.
18.	Generic name	14. One of the primary alerts for identifying extreme adverse drug reactions discovered during and after the review process.
25.	Adherence	15. A physiologic or psychologic need for a substance.
13.	Combination drug	16. Agents naturally produced in animal cells, by microorganisms, or by the body itself.
4.	Pharmacologic classification	17. Method of organizing drugs is based on their therapeutic usefulness in treating particular diseases or disorders.
14.	Black box warnings	18. Less complicated and easier to remember than chemical names.
15.	Dependence	19. Physical signs of discomfort.
30.	Adverse effect	20. Refers to how a medicine changes the body.
33.	Potency	21. Nontherapeutic reaction to a drug.
28.	Maintenance doses	22. A severe type of allergic reaction that involves the massive, systemic release of histamine and other chemical mediators of inflammation that can lead to life-threatening shock.
6.	Therapeutic	23. The study of drug movement throughout the body.
21.	Side effect	24. Occurs when the medication has reached its highest concentration in the bloodstream.
16.	Biologics	25. Taking a medication in the manner prescribed by the health care provider or, in the case of OTC drugs, following the instructions on the label.
29.	Onset of drug action	26. Amount of time a drug maintains its therapeutic effect.
1.	Drug	27. A higher amount of drug often given only once or twice to "prime" the bloodstream with a sufficient level of drug.
32.	Idiosyncratic responses	28. Given to keep the plasma drug concentration in the therapeutic range.

27.	Loading dose	29. Represents the amount of time it takes to produce a therapeutic effect after drug administration.
34.	Allergic reaction	30. An unfavorable drug reaction.
20.	Pharmacodynamics	31. The magnitude of maximal response that can be produced from a particular drug.
31.	Efficacy	32. Unpredictable and unexplained drug reactions.
9.	Trade name	33. Will produce a therapeutic effect at a lower dose, compared with another drug in the same class.
19.	Withdrawal	34. Acquired hyper-response of body defenses to a foreign substance (allergen).
5.	Pharmacogenetics	35. How a drug produces its physiologic effect in the body.
2.	Teratogen	36. Desirable effects.

Key to Section II

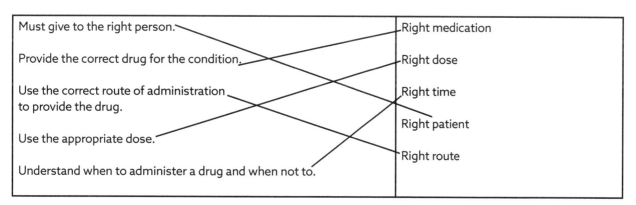

Must give to the right person.	Right medication
Provide the correct drug for the condition.	Right dose
Use the correct route of administration to provide the drug.	Right time
Use the appropriate dose.	Right patient
Understand when to administer a drug and when not to.	Right route

Key to Section V

Dependence	The patient has an intense desire continue to use the drug.
Physical dependence	A need for a drug, either physical or physiologic.
Withdrawal	Occurs with the repeated use of a drug; patient's physical condition adapts to the drug.
Psychological dependence	When drug is no longer available, the patient experiences discomfort.

Answers to Critical Thinking Questions

1. **A, C, D, E.** Baseline vital signs, following the five rights, answering any of the patient's questions, and assessing for reactions are the nurse's responsibility. Accurate health care provider orders are a part of ensuring safe medication administration and the prescriber is responsible for accuracy of the order.

2. **A, C. D.** The nurse should make sure the allergy is documented on the chart, the health care provider is notified, and a medi-alert bracelet is placed on the patient.

3. **B.** STAT means that the medication should be given immediately and 5 min or less is when the medication should be given.

4. **B.** The nurse should contact the health care provider to verify the NPO order and if the patient should take the medication.

5. **D.** Chronic kidney failure increases the amount of time of the medication's action due to decreased excretion, so it is important to monitor for any drug toxicity.

6. **B, C.** The patient needs to be assessed for possible reactions to the wrong medication being administered, and the nurse manager should be notified. An incidence report is filled out but it is not to be put in the chart or documented in the chart. The risk management team will follow-up after the incidence report is submitted.

7. **B.** It is important for the nurse to always validate and reassure the patient by checking the orders and then teach the patient about h the medication.

8. **D.** Giving a loading dose is done to make sure the medication achieves the therapeutic range more rapidly, followed by the maintenance dose.

Reference: Adams, M. P., Holland, N., & Urban, C. Q. (2019). *Pharmacology for nurses* (6th ed.). Pearson Education USA. https://bookshelf.vitalsource.com/books/9780135268438